the little book of dirty diet tricks

365 WAYS TO LOSE WEIGHT

OR LOOK LIKE YOU DID

WITHOUT LOSING YOUR

MIND ALONG THE WAY

THREE RIVERS PRESS • NEW YORK

the little book of dirty diet tricks

CAROLE BODGER

Published by Three Rivers Press, New York, New York. Member of the Crown Publishing Group, a division of Random House, Inc.

www.randomhouse.com

THREE RIVERS PRESS and the Tugboat design are registered trademarks of Random House, Inc.

Printed in the United States of America

DESIGN BY ELINA D. NUDELMAN

Library of Congress Cataloging-in-Publication Data

Bodger, Carole.
   The little book of dirty diet tricks : 365 ways to lose weight or look like you did without losing your mind along the way / by Carole Bodger.—1st ed.
       p. cm.
1. Weight loss.
   [DNLM: 1. Diet, Reducing—Popular Works. 2. Obesity—prevention & control—Popular Works. 3. Weight Loss—Popular Works. WD 212 B666L 2002] I. Title
   RM222.2 B5895 2002
   613.2'5—dc21   2002001249

ISBN 0-609-80925-3

10 9 8 7 6 5 4 3 2 1

First Edition

To Edwin Bon, for loving me through thick and thin

Acknowledgments

Beautiful women and men of all sizes contributed in so very many ways to this book, and I thank them from the bottom of my heart. Special love and gratitude to Tamar Arnon, Nancy Guimond, Sharon Miller, Steve Ricci, Deva Skiles, Ellen Stock, and Robin Ward for unwavering support and friendship sweeter than all the chocolate in the world; to my dear husband, Ed Bon, for the feast that is our life; to my agent, Liza Dawson, for so generously nourishing my dream; to my editor and friend, Shaye Areheart, for making this the most delicious editorial experience an author could hope to have. And to Lorrie Bodger, whose encouragement, guidance, and friendship have enriched my life beyond expression, I cannot give thanks enough.

—C.B.
Atlanta, Georgia

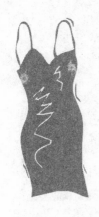
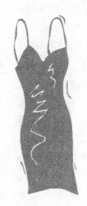
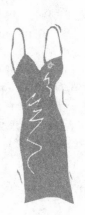

"How many pounds did *you* lose?"

It's one of the first questions I get asked in my line of work. My answer is the same one you might hear from any other woman who has lost—and found (and lost and found)—weight on the many diets we've seen come and go through the years: "Hundreds."

We are not alone. More than 97 million men and women—over half the adult U.S. population—are overweight, according to the National Institutes of Health, and of the fifty-million-plus Americans who will go on weight-loss diets this year, only 5 percent, the Federal Trade Commission says, will keep the weight off. They are housewives and executives, teachers and technicians, flight attendants and postal workers . . . even health and fitness writers. We fight a common, and ongoing, battle: the battle of the bulge.

The last time I gained weight was when I left my job at a magazine's editorial offices to work from home, with my new coworkers, Ben and Jerry. And Edy. And Sara Lee. Forty pounds later, having sworn not to purchase a stitch of clothing in yet a larger size, I was about to launder the very last pair of jeans whose stitches could still hold me. As I reached for the detergent I was struck by the realization that if I put those jeans into the washer and dryer, exposing them to shrinkage of as much as a micron, I would never get them back on my body again. The jeans didn't get washed that day, but I cleaned up my weight-loss act. I started fighting dirty.

Like many women, I, too, have eaten my way through the Cottage Cheese/Jell-O/Tuna Salad Age (extra lettuce, please), to the bacon cheeseburgers of the Atkins Era (hold the lettuce, please). I even confess to guiltily slinking into the local pharmacy for a bottle of syrup of ipecac during a regrettable binge-purge phase. I know what it's like to throw an entire bag of cookies into the trash only to "rescue" them when no one is looking, to divide a portion in half—and then eat both halves. I understand that when it comes to overeating, "*just* say no" just won't cut it.

Another thing that won't cut it: patience. So what if every health professional worth her protein—including me, a health and fitness writer for many years—knows that nothing but slow-and-steady weight loss is either healthy or sustainable. I, like every other dieter, wanted to lose it all *now*. If my body wouldn't cooperate, my closet would have to help me look as though it had. A few wardrobe adjustments, a lot of black ensembles, some makeup and hair tricks, and a little bit of strategic posturing, and at least some of those pounds were instantly "gone."

That's what I'd like to help you to do: not just lose weight, but look like you did, right away.

Losing weight is hard work that calls for changing everything from our behavior (what we eat, how we eat it, how we work it off) to the beliefs we've been spoon-fed since childhood (food is love, children will starve in

Africa if we don't clean our plates, a cookie will make everything all right).

Like a drug, food can be addictive, but we cannot go cold turkey (pardon the expression), or put on a patch and quit. Not if we plan to continue living and breathing, anyway. We sit down to the table with it (if not stand over the sink with it) several times a day; we encounter it in social and business settings; we receive it as a gift. We are seduced by its image in magazines and on television, and have to fend off its advances from friends and family eager to fill us with everything from get-well casseroles to seductive Valentine Godiva chocolates. Food pushers are everywhere—even Girl Scouts show up with it at our door, beseeching us to buy.

Beyond diet and exercise alone, weight loss involves self-motivation, patience, perseverance, willpower, the occasional gnashing of teeth, and a sense of humor to get us through it without throwing up our hands and diving headlong into the Häagen-Dazs. It involves cooking strategies, food-shopping strategies, get-off-the-couch strategies, restaurant strategies, home-alone-with-the-refrigerator strategies, surviving-the-holidays-with-the-family strategies, and vacation strategies, to name a few. Most important, long-lasting success means never feeling deprived, but being able to live life to its fullest—complete with parties, vacations, dinners out, and holiday celebrations, even wearing swimsuits!—just like "regular people" do. Weight loss is a fight to have your food *and* have fun; to have your cake and eat it. I say there's no reason why you can't.

This book wasn't written to advance lengthy arguments about the importance of good nutrition or the benefits of physical activity. These are things you already know. Neither will it put you on a diet or prescribe a program of exercise. There are many other good publications to do that. As someone who has not only read extensively on these very topics, but written as extensively about them, I learned that to practice what is preached calls for more than believing it is important, or even that it works. It calls for food warfare: what I call "dirty tricks."

And that brings us to what this book *will* give you: a shoot-from-the-hip, take-no-prisoners guide to everything the nutrition and exercise gurus won't tell you fast enough—from how to cut fat and calories without feeling like you've cut out your taste buds, to exorcising the fear of exercise, to Restaurant Dining 101 (Repeat after me: "Please remove the bread basket from the table"). It's about helping you learn how to stick to your diet and exercise programs, and how to keep your sanity while you do. Never mind the way you're supposed to behave (have a little sliver of the pie), this book addresses the way you (and I) *do* behave (finish off the rest of the pie after everyone else has gone to bed), and helps you change that behavior, one pie at a time.

Because losing weight can seem an endless journey, these pages offer strategies to shorten the trip by helping you look thinner along the way. You'll find clothing and makeup techniques, posture and hairstyling tips—even the way you decorate your home can help. Who wants to wait until she *is* slim to *look* slim? This book will show you how.

My goal: to serve you a year's worth of the sanest, healthiest, and best weight-loss and look-slim strategies there are; a tasty assortment of tried-and-true basics in bite-size servings that are fun to read, easy to do, and that work—whether you are outright heavy, unpleasantly plump, or just want to take off the five pounds you gained on your last vacation. The tips will work as well for gourmet cooks as for heat-and-servers, for the physically active and the sofa-bound. Above all, they're designed for people who might know better but aren't always able to "just do it." In other words, they work for human beings.

I love food, and I eat a lot of it; I abhor exercise, but I keep moving; the word "diet" makes me hungry, but I lost—and kept off—all the weight I wanted gone. I fought dirty and I won the battle. So can you.

Key

 Dining and Diet

 Looking Slimmer

 Exercise and Physical Activity

 Behavior Changes and Mind Games

 Restaurant Dining

 Tools and Products

 Travel

 Liquor and Spirits

 Holidays and Special Events

the little book of dirty diet tricks

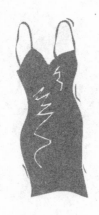
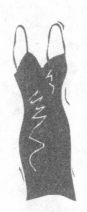
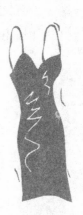

1

Wear black. The little black dress—or pants, or sweater, or blouse—will make you look littler. *Nothing* works better. But if we *do* find a darker color, we'll let you know.

2

Don't eat while you're standing. No, the calories don't travel down to and out of the soles of your feet—they just travel faster into your mouth because you're telling yourself the food doesn't count. And yes, the extra food you consume more than outstrips your barely-elevated-because-you're-standing metabolic rate. Eat only while you're seated at a proper table.

3

Before going to a restaurant, stand before the mirror and say the words, "Please remove the bread basket from the table." There. Now you know you can actually make those words come from your very own mouth. Say them to the waiter when the bread basket arrives.

4

Use your hand as a portion guide. Don't eat more than a palm's worth of anything.

5

Eat with chopsticks to slow yourself down—at least until you're so good with them that they don't. Then try holding your utensils in your other hand.

6

Lose the TV and stereo remotes—on purpose. Get up and change those channels and stations yourself.

7

TIP OF THE WEEK　　　**USE MORE THAN ONE "SCALE."**

There are many more gauges of success than the numbers on the bathroom scale: the number of stairs you can run up without getting winded, your clothing size, the belt notch you use, the compliments you get. And then there are your measurements: With muscle weighing more than fat, you might be getting thinner (and better toned), even though your weight is staying the same. So count those stairs, monitor your dress size, watch your belt notch, count those compliments, and measure away! Not all of these will change or occur as swiftly as the changes you measure in pounds, but each is a definite gauge of progress worth noting in an "I Did It!" journal—and celebrating. Thinner thighs, a smaller size, pockets into which you can actually *put* things—all are sure signs of success. Set lots of goals, and reward yourself whenever you reach one.

8

Listen to your corduroys. Don't think about wearing them until your thighs don't make that sound when you walk. And if they're wide wale corduroys, think long and hard.

9

Get a gum-ball bank. When having just one of anything is a challenge, per-portion payments can help. Fill it with sugar-free gum balls, jelly beans, or other low-calorie treats, and put the money toward a new something in a smaller size.

10

 Replace an Oreo with a Fig Newton. With about the same calories per cookie, the Oreo contains $2\frac{1}{3}$ grams of fat, the Newton contains $1\frac{1}{4}$ grams of fat. You do the math.

11

 When you walk, swing your arms. Involve more of your body to get more of a workout.

12

 Do a "Miss America." Stand at an angle that presents a three-quarter body profile.

13

 Establish an end-of-meal routine—a walk around the block, a relaxing session of needlework, reading a chapter of a book—to let you know that eating time is over.

If you do, you won't succumb to the urge to buy out the entire store or to climb bodily into the frozen desserts section in an effort to "become one" with Ben and Jerry. If you can't eat before you get to the grocery, and the sight of all that food is making you ravenous, head straight for the produce section and tear into a package of prewashed baby carrots. Chomp as many as it takes to satisfy your hunger during the rest of the visit. (And no, the cashier won't mind ringing up the price of the empty carrot bag.)

15

To avoid supermarket temptations entirely, make a sensible shopping list and send another family member out to shop. Can't depend on your spouse or teen to follow the list? Use the market's customer service or an Internet service to do the job.

16

Weigh weekly, measure monthly. For a good record of your progress, weigh yourself on a good, no-kidding-yourself digital scale weekly, not daily, to keep daily fluctuations from giving a false sense of what's what. Take measurements of your hips, waist, bust, upper thighs, and upper arms monthly, not weekly. Lost inches don't show up as quickly as lost pounds. Why measure both? Since muscle weighs more than fat (it's about three times the density), you might be getting thinner (and better toned) even though your weight is staying the same. Take credit wherever you can.

17

Tape a picture of your skinny self to the refrigerator for inspiration. Remind yourself what you *can* look like.

18

Tape a picture of your fat self to the refrigerator for motivation. Remind yourself what you *don't want* to look like.

19

Never wear anklets. Ever. We're not talking about the athletic socks that protect and support your feet during workouts, but those awful little-girl things that come back into style every few years just for spite. They make your legs appear shorter and wider. Not to mention what they'll do to your reputation for being someone who has good taste.

20

Wear high heels for a tall, slim look. For an even longer-legged look, choose deep V-shaped or low-scooped pumps.

21

Foods can be misleading. Many of those that have gained a reputation for being low calorie or low fat aren't as low as you might expect, so check labels. Cottage cheese, the long-reigning Queen of Diet Food, is available in many versions, from nonfat to 4 percent and higher. Yogurt can contain as much as seven grams of fat or more in the average eight-ounce serving (one popular variety, with 280 calories and ten grams of fat, contains seventy more calories and as much fat as you'd find in a small order of McDonald's french fries). Even low-fat yogurt is allowed to contain one to six grams of fat. And it doesn't always depend on flavor: one brand's lightest line contains 120 calories and no fat, whether vanilla, white chocolate raspberry, or crème caramel.

Other foods worth checking:

- *Tofu and other soy products:* Innocent looking, but high in fat.

- *Edamame:* They're green, and they're beans, but they are not green beans; they are soybeans. See above.

- *Diet shakes and drinks:* Intended as meal replacements, most are fortified with more calories than you'd consume in a good-size sandwich and a salad.

- *Fruit drinks and flavored seltzers:* Check the labels for added sugar.

22

Eat at an expensive restaurant. The kitchen is usually far more accommodating when it comes to special dietary requests. The serving sizes are usually smaller. And you won't be able to afford as much food, anyway.

23

Don't keep up with the Joneses. Take one bite of food for every two your dining companion takes (or, if your companion is a speed eater, take one bite for every three). When she lets the waiter remove her plate, let him take yours along with it.

24

If you're dining out and *must* have dessert, convince your companion to order a serving for him- or herself, and to let you have a single fork- or spoonful. Warning: to be attempted with only the most supportive companions.

25

Use secrets for success. More than one diet-conscious homemaker has been known to covertly replace the family's whole milk with lower-fat milk, and to replace the salt with light salt. What the others didn't know didn't hurt them; in fact, it was better for their health. And with a gradual switchover, nobody's taste buds could tell. Not that *we* would ever consider doing such a sneaky thing . . .

26

When you make a sandwich, replace one slice of bread with a fresh vegetable "topper." A couple of big fresh lettuce leaves or a slice of bell pepper will serve nicely.

"Boost" your sandwiches with lettuce, tomato, sprouts, cucumber slices, bell peppers, and other fresh vegetables. Along with the bigger crunch, you'll get a bigger sandwich with few additional calories and no extra fat.

28

| TIP OF THE WEEK | MAKE A WARDROBE POISON LIST. |

If you want to look slim, there are some things you should just never wear. Ever.

Cable-knit fisherman's sweaters

Denim skirts

Capri pants

Hip-huggers

Trench coats, safari jackets, and anything else bedecked with wide belts, giant pockets, epaulets, and huge lapels

Muumuus

Large patterns

Horizontal patterns

Shiny fabrics

Stiff fabrics

Furry, fuzzy fabrics

Ruffles

Solid expanses of white, or "hot" or "electric" colors

Clunky, chunky platform shoes

Shoes with straps around the ankle or instep

White shoes (no matter *what* time of year)

Anklets

Tight clothing

Big, round accessories, including earrings, necklaces, buttons, and belt buckles

29

Wear vertical stripes. Patterns that move the eye up and down rather than side to side emphasize your height instead of your width. The exceptions: wide vertical stripes, which can make even a thin person look like a circus tent; and vertical stripes on clingy clothing or hosiery, which can highlight bumps and bulges you didn't even know you had.

30

Choose tailored garments. The hide-all diaphanous look will only add the inches you want to take away.

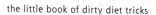

TIP
OF THE
MONTH

"STAY IN THE CAR."

Think of your efforts to reach your weight goal as a car trip. For some, it might be a drive across town, for others it's a cross-country trek; but for everyone—wherever the starting point, and whatever the chosen destination—a journey lies ahead. Expect some red lights and stop signs along the way, and remember: They don't mean the trip is over; they're just part of the ride.

And like all car trips, it can present unexpected surprises. Have you ever gotten lost? Had to take a detour? Run out of gas? Become stuck in traffic? Did you just get out of the car and give up? Not if you wanted to get where you were going. You asked for directions, turned the car around, refueled, waited out the jam. The trip might have taken longer than you wanted or expected, it might have taken you on a different route than you originally planned, but as long as you stayed in the car, you eventually did arrive. When it comes to weight loss, the same rules of the road apply.

Never lose sight of your destination, the reason you set out on the journey, or the benefits of arriving. For smoother traveling, anticipate your personal detours, where you might need to yield, when you'll need to "fill up," whom you can turn to for help. Map out a plan and, most important of all, *keep driving!*

Scenic overlooks and side trips: Stopping every now and then to take in a gorgeous view or visit an historic sight can make a journey more enjoyable; in fact, it might be the only way to endure longer rides. It will delay your arrival, but without it you might not be able to tolerate the trip at all. Think of no-holds-barred celebratory dinners and big pieces of birthday cake in the same way. Enjoy them and move on.

Speed limits: Some of us are driving Corvettes and others are cruising along in Ol' Betsy, but we all have to follow the rules of the road. The highway system imposes speed limits for your protection, and so does the body—there's only so much weight per week you can lose safely, and in a way that will stay off. Trying to rush the safety rate by starving yourself (ever wonder why it's called *fasting?*) will only backfire as your body, deprived of the fuel it needs, slows the metabolism to conserve energy and survive. *Crash* diets, like any other kind of crash, do nothing but harm.

Tolls: No matter where you're going, there are costs involved (tolls, gasoline, the time spent on the trip), and the same applies to your weight-loss journey. The more desirable the destination, the less you will begrudge the "expense." Paying the price—by forgoing a dessert, planning meals in advance, being more physically active than you might feel like being—is easier if you remember how great you'll feel and look when you arrive.

32

As Valentine's Day approaches, tell Cupid to tell your sweetheart you prefer your confections to be rich in karats, not calories. Better yet, bat your eyelashes ever so sweetly and—in no uncertain terms—tell him yourself.

33

Of course, you're not *really* going to complain about receiving a heart-shaped box of chocolates from your beloved on Valentine's Day, but that doesn't mean you have to eat it. Exchange the sweets for a kiss. No, not Hershey's. Then lovingly toss the chocolates into the trash when he's not looking.

34

Do "traffic-light isometrics" on the road. While you're waiting for the light to change, strengthen and tone your stomach or buttock muscles by clenching and then relaxing them. Stopped in a traffic jam? Keep one foot on the brake and use the other to "write the alphabet" (rotate your foot to "write" each letter), or do a few heel lifts (press down on the toes for a few seconds while lifting the heel) to shape calves. If you're the passenger, do them while you're riding across bridges, through tunnels, or from one highway exit to the next. Facial isometrics can help tighten chin and neck, but are too easily mistaken for road rage. Save them to do at home.

35

 The more beautiful the cake, the less likely you'll be to "start the party" early, if you know what we mean. And beauty doesn't have to mean high-calorie—many adornments are as easy on your waist as they are on your eyes. Other boons: They're great for marking portion sizes around a cake's circumference, and are just as good-looking on one-serving cupcakes and tarts:

- Strawberries and other berries, halved or whole

- Mandarin orange slices, drained and dried

- Banana slices

- Jelly beans

- Coconut "grass" (reduced-fat coconut shreds, tossed with a few drops of green food coloring)

- Pineapple butterflies (well-drained canned pineapple slice "wings" and a halved cherry "body")

- Dried fruit (raisins, currants, apricot slivers or bits, sliced dates)

- Grape halves

- Thin slices of orange or lemon

- Slivers of orange or lemon peel (peel the fruit thinly with a vegetable peeler, and cut the strips into slivers with scissors)

- Raisins (purple and yellow)

- A light sprinkling of sprinkles, or colored dots

- Inedible decorations, including fresh flowers and leaves, parasols, ribbons

- Practically inedible decorations, such as dragées—silver, gold, or colored "beads" that are technically edible, but only at the risk of cracking your teeth

36

Give yourself a manicure when a food craving strikes, applying extra layers of slow-drying nail polish. It will make your hands look prettier, and keep them occupied and out of trouble (i.e., food containers) until the craving fades.

37

Take a shower or bath when a food craving strikes. It will relax you, and keep your whole body occupied and out of trouble (i.e., the kitchen) until the craving fades.

38

Phone a talkative friend when a food craving strikes. Call from a phone *with* a cord that's *outside* the kitchen, and stay on until the craving fades.

39

Go for a walk when a food craving strikes. It will work off some calories, and keep you out of trouble until the craving fades. (Avoid walks anywhere near a grocery until it does.)

40

Go monochrome. For instant taller and thinner: pick a color; pick any dark color. Then dress yourself in it from top to bottom to create an unbroken vertical (read *slimming*) line. For interest, contrast different fabrics and weaves (a black wool skirt with a black cashmere sweater, and a black leather handbag). For a variation on the theme, wear a variety of same-"weight" colors (violet, crimson, and navy), or wear one color in slightly different shades (mahogany, chocolate, and coffee).

41

Purge your wardrobe of all clothing that contains an expanse of bright yellow, or any color that even remotely brings to mind the word "hot" (hot pink) or "electric" (electric orange). There is a reason why warning signs appear in these colors. Observe the proper level of alarm.

42

TIP OF THE WEEK	INSTEAD OF A LUNCH (OR DINNER) DATE WITH YOUR FRIEND, MAKE A DATE TO DO SOMETHING TOGETHER THAT ISN'T BASED AROUND FOOD.

Satisfy your hunger by having a light meal before you meet, and enjoy the companionship without the calories. (Note: You can also make these dates with *yourself*.)

- Visit a museum

- Shop

- Window shop

- Take a walk

- Get a manicure or pedicure together

- Get a makeup demonstration together

- Go to the park, and feed some pigeons instead of yourselves (feed them something that doesn't tempt *you*)

43

Don't clean your plate. Always leave something over. Tell Mom you'll send a financial contribution to help those poor children starving in Africa, and throw the remainder of your meal into the trash, or a suitable container.

44

Have someone else clear the table to keep you from being tempted by leftovers.

45

Brush your teeth, floss, gargle with mouthwash, or chew a stick of sugarless gum immediately after your meal to stop yourself from eating more.

46

Keep your light on the inside. For a longer, leaner look, wear light-color accents away from your outlines. Letting a bright blouse peep from inside a jacket, or dangling a light flowing scarf down your middle, for instance, will create a vertical line that brings the focus to your face.

47

Don't "eat and." Don't eat and read, don't eat and watch television, don't eat and work, don't eat and talk on the telephone. . . . If you eat at the same time something else is demanding your attention, you won't be able to appreciate the food, or notice how much of it you're consuming. Apply your full concentration to eating when you eat, and the meal or snack will be more satisfying.

48

Play soft, slow background music during meals. It slows your pace, and it's good for your digestion.

49

TIP OF THE WEEK	SATISFY THY CRAVINGS.

You *can* crave your cake and eat it, too—as long as you're prepared with the right kind of cake. Cravings, by definition, are powerful urges that strike when you least expect them. Think of them as the guerrilla-warfare food group: sneaky and relentless. Fight back with the same ammunition that's coming your way: By stocking your refrigerator and pantry with lower-calorie, lower-fat versions of the foods in each of the craving groups—sweet, salty, crunchy, creamy, and choco-late—you can satisfy your desire without sabo-taging your diet.

Is the pint of high-test, chocolate-chocolate-fudge-swirl ice cream that your partner put in the freezer calling your name? Reach for the supply of low-calorie fudgsicles you stocked alongside it. Craving some crunch? Grab the snack-size bag of baked chips you've hidden in the pantry. Remember: A craving for chocolate, or crunch, can't be quelled by a peach—or ten peaches—and denying your desire will backfire when you try answering your need for a little of "this" with a *lot* of "that" (i.e., ten peaches, *and* the chocolate, *and* the chips). Be prepared.

50

Don't buy anything that's labeled "family size" if you want to keep from becoming family-size.

51

Decorate your house with big furniture. You'll look smaller when you're sitting on or standing next to it.

52

Stand near fatter people. They make you look thinner.

53

Count your calories. Aloud. Before you eat something, find out how many calories it contains and count out the full number—slowly—before you put it into your mouth. The delay will allow you the chance to fully grasp what you're about to do, to change your mind, and will slow your progress toward second helpings. If you're considering a Snickers, with 280 calories in a two-ounce bar, you can use all the extra minutes you can to start working it off.

54

Enjoy a Blue Moon Treat. Special event "eating occasions"—like birthdays and anniversaries—can be celebrated with the occasional splurge. But remember: Even if you *can* convince yourself that *your* birthday cake has no calories, the argument won't work on other people's cakes, too.

Fake olives. Save the liquid from a jar of olives, and use it to immerse the contents of a jar of mushrooms for a day or so. Voilà! "Olives" without the calories or fat.

TIP OF THE WEEK	ORDER YOUR PIZZA YOUR WAY.

Admit it: There are times when nothing else will do. Happily, there are many ways to minimize the potential diet damage of this home delivery favorite.

- Order the pie plain and, while you're waiting for it to arrive, prepare your own fresh or steamed toppings, which are almost guaranteed to be lower calorie and lower fat than the bathed-in-butter ingredients pizzerias typically use. Consider mushrooms, red and green peppers, zucchini, broccoli, onions, jalapeños, spinach, capers, even a sprinkling of reduced-fat cheese shreds or light Parmesan. Accompany with a big, satisfying salad.

- Request thin crust.

- If your pizza-eating companions want to heap on the calories, order a "half and half" pie, and keep the calories heaped on their half.

- Ask the pizzeria to slice your pie into half-size slices.

- When the pizza arrives, sop up excess oil with a paper towel, pressing down on the top of the pie and repeating to absorb as much as you can, before adding toppings.

- After arranging your toppings on the pizza—but before you start to eat—remove the number of slices you plan to have, wrap the remainder in individual portions, and stow them in the freezer.

57

Boycott the big and the round. Replace large, round jewelry (such as big beaded necklaces and earrings) with slim and simple elegance. Replace large, round shiny buttons with smaller, sleeker styles that match the fabric they're buttoning. Ditto: belt buckles. "Rotund" is not a shape with which you want to associate.

58

Use a little fat to fight your fat. Besides being essential for health, small amounts of dietary fat can help you to feel fuller longer without endangering your diet. Emphasis on the word "small."

You weigh yourself every week, and most every week the numbers are (hooray!) smaller. But no matter how hard you look, that quarter of a pound—or even two or three pounds—just doesn't immediately appear in the mirror. Not seeing visible signs of accomplishment can be discouraging to even the most successful dieter. But keep a detailed bar or line graph of your weight, and even the smallest loss will show as success. Here's how:

Step 1. On a sheet of graph paper, draw a vertical line, or axis, along the left side, and a horizontal axis across the bottom.

Step 2. Write a range of weights along the vertical axis. Try half- or quarter-pound increments, with your current weight toward the top of the sheet (allowing lots of room to lose).

Step 3. Write the dates you weigh yourself (preferably weekly, to spare yourself the frustration of daily fluctuations) along the horizontal axis.

Step 4. Draw a bold red line across all the weights ending in the numeral 0 (150, 160, 170, etc.), and a bold green line across all the weights ending in the numeral 5 (155, 165, 175, etc.).

Step 5. Every time you weigh yourself, record the results on your chart, and enjoy the visible signs of your success. And if you do take an upturn now and then, look back to your starting point, acknowledge how far you've come, and be reinspired.

Use your weight chart to set—and reach—small, doable goals. Look upon those red and green horizons as "mini finish lines." Forget about the ultimate number of pounds you feel you need to lose, and aim for the next red or green milestone on your graph. When you reach one, celebrate, recharge your engines, and set out for the next.

60

Display fruits and vegetables at eye level and within easy reach in your refrigerator's prime space. Keep a good supply prewashed, peeled, sliced, and ready to eat for emergency munchy attacks.

61

Use your refrigerator's fruit and vegetable bins to hide any temptations your family members insist on having in the house. The back of your pantry's hard-to-reach top shelf is another option, as is that unfathomable "mystery cabinet" over the fridge. Out of sight (and reach), less likely to be in mind. Or mouth.

62

Get the person who brought those temptations home to hide them himself. Don't ask where.

63

Makeup matters. Like the colors of your wardrobe, the colors in your makeup palette, and how they're applied, can make a big difference in how round or slim you look. Draw attention to your eyes with dark neutral shadow, mascara, and liner in deep browns or grays; opt for a lighter neutral lipstick, keeping the focus away from heavy chins. Blend foundation to prevent lines of demarcation from emphasizing chins and wattles; narrow full cheeks with a hint of blusher just under the cheekbone and along the sides of your face. Apply your makeup like an artist, and check it often. Better yet, have a professional makeup artist apply it and teach you how. You'll look great, feel like a million bucks, and be more likely to treat yourself accordingly.

64

To add length to round faces, part hair on the side, in a silky straight down do, or in an upsweep.

Keep bangs on the wispy side, if you wear them, to avoid a face-broadening horizontal line.

65

Watch your lines. Vertical lines—in fabric patterns, in the way your clothing drapes, in the way a garment is cut, in the shape of your neckline, in the direction your jewelry falls, even in the direction in which your shoe tops lead the eye—will make you look taller and slimmer. Horizontals—hemlines, necklines, waistlines—do the opposite. Worse, the eye moves more slowly over horizontal lines, making them all the more powerful.

66

Wear skirts that go with the flow. Boxes aren't flattering. Neither are teepees. The most slimming skirts are longer, in flowing fabrics that don't stand out from the body. Denim skirts, this does not mean you.

67

Wear finer weaves of fabric. Fabrics stiff enough to stand on their own tend to stand away from your body. The result: a bigger-looking body. They also tend to hold creases, emphasizing your widest areas as though they're underlined. Wool, cotton, linen, silk, synthetics, and synthetic blends can all be processed in ways that are more or less slimming; look for those that flow and drape into vertical folds. The finer the weave, the better the drape. The better the drape, the better you look. Hold the garment at arm's length and move it from side to side. If it doesn't sway and fold a little, put it back on the rack.

68

Walk for a cause. Sign up for a fund-raising walk-a-thon or bike-a-thon to help out a cause dear to your heart. For extra motivation, enlist sponsors who will contribute by the mile. Good for your body, good for your soul, good for us all!

69

Computer-enhance a photo of yourself to see how great you'll look when you're slim. Never mind liposuction: Today's computer technology lets you delete double chins and narrow your waistline with the touch of a keystroke. Print out two copies of the image—one for the refrigerator door and one for your purse.

TIP OF THE WEEK	B.Y.O.S.

 Bring your own snacks—wherever you go—to keep yourself from diving like a kamikaze pilot out of your good intentions and into the diet suicide of fattening fast-food restaurant and convenience store choices. Having a healthy snack at the first rumbling of your stomach will help stave off the hunger that makes you a calorie-attracting magnet. It will allow you to actually bypass the Mrs. Fields kiosk at the shopping mall and will (yes, really) reduce food cravings. Dried fruits, rice cakes, low-calorie nutrition bars, fruits, and even snack packs of fat-free pretzels or air-popped popcorn are some of the many good portables that will easily fit into your purse.

71

 Bring your own diet salad dressing to restaurants that might have a limited selection (or none) of their own. Purse-size packets are available in the diet-food aisles of many supermarkets.

72

 Instead of a sit-down lunch, visit a local green market and "sample." Walk around between tastes.

73

Bring your lunch to work. You'll save money *and* calories. A good thermal lunch bag and a few freezable cold packs will get you and your comestibles to the office, through lunch, and safely through an afternoon snack. (Take *that*, Office Doughnut Boy.)

74

Chew sugarless gum while you prepare meals. It'll keep you from tasting (a.k.a. eating) that extra serving's worth.

75

When you cook or bake, keep a bowl of water nearby in which to drop utensils as soon as you're done using them, to keep you from licking them clean.

76

When you prepare dinner, securely wrap anything more than one portion of the meal, and stash it in the freezer *before* you sit down to eat. You'll be less inclined to have seconds. Or thirds.

TIP OF THE **WEEK**   **MAKE YOUR SOUP EAT LIKE A MEAL.**

Bulk up your soup with veggies—carrots, mushrooms, green beans, and other low-calorie, low-fat ingredients—and it will become a filling course on its own. For a quick fix, buy the frozen, mixed variety (broccoli, cauliflower, and carrots are among the lowest calorie combos), toss half the package into a pot of canned soup, and heat together. For a richer taste, start by draining all but the stock from the soup, add the frozen veggies to the stock, heat for a few minutes, then return the ingredients you removed and continue heating. Add spices and seasonings as desired.

78

Run from chunky, clunky, and high-cut footwear. Put as much distance as possible between you and platform or extended-sole styles, shoes with high vamps that cut horizontally across the foot, and those with straps around the ankle or across the instep. All will make your leg look heavier. Look for V-shaped or low-scoop designs, and slimming silhouettes.

79

Match your shoe style to your foot style. If your ankle is on the sturdy side, step away from fragile-looking shoes, like strappy sandals and stilettos, which will make your ankle look even sturdier in contrast. Alternatively, don't let delicate tootsies be overwhelmed by heavy footwear.

80

Hide "shorty" or mid-calf boots beneath slacks. Unless you have a pant leg covering them, they'll draw a look-wider horizontal line right across the part of your lower leg that is the heaviest.

81

Empty your wardrobe of pockets. Even if you don't have anything in them, they will look like you do.

82

Match your lingerie to your bedsheets. You'll blend.

83

Carry a purse-size calorie counter to use discreetly when you're out to eat, visiting, or traveling.

84

RESEARCH RESTAURANTS BEFORE YOU GO.

Knowing what to order *before* you arrive at a restaurant can make a difference weighable in pounds. Happily, more and more eateries are making their menus available on the Internet, and many national chains include nutritional information as well. (Some independent websites even have interactive programs with which you can enter the name of a restaurant, along with the maximum number of calories, fat, cholesterol, or sodium you want in your meal, and learn the menu items that meet your requirements. Search the Internet for "restaurant calories" and similar phrases.)

If you can't find the menu in cyberspace, ask to have it mailed or faxed; at the very least, you can pick one up at the restaurant a day or so before your meal. By having the information in advance, you can target the least fattening selections, decide on your order, and not be tempted by another look at the menu when you arrive.

85

Enjoy a light salad or bowl of soup before you go out to eat to take the edge off your hunger. It will help keep you from overordering, ordering unwisely, or consuming the entire bread basket— wicker and all—while you wait for your meal to arrive.

86

Eat with someone whom you want to impress with your slow and gracious table manners.

87

Buy small wineglasses. Yes, the size and shape of the glass is important to connoisseurs judging the quality, aroma, and "personality" of the wine or other spirit, but for our purposes the smaller the glass, the better the glass. True friends will love you even if you use tiny dessert glasses.

88

Choose between dessert wine and dessert. A four-ounce glass of dessert wine averages about 185 calories, more than you'd find in some brownies.

89

Avoid "umbrella drinks." If it comes with an umbrella, an oversize swizzle stick, a sparkler, or has any other sort of ornamental flourish springing from the rim, you can be sure it also comes with extra calories.

90

JOIN A GYM—AND GO.

Sorry, but paying annual dues alone isn't enough. As much as you want to believe your membership pass is a mystical talisman capable of magically transforming your body into a model of fitness and health, the only way the pass will work is if you use it to enter the facility and take advantage of the equipment, the trainers, the classes, and the motivational support available inside.

• Choose a gym that's easy to get to, close to either your home or workplace, with hours that suit yours. Leave yourself no excuse.

• Look for a facility whose personal trainers are certified by a nationally recognized certifying agency; look for initials such as ACSM (American College of Sports Medicine) or ACE (American Council on Exercise) after their names. An educational background in health and fitness, and CPR training, are definite pluses; and friendly, helpful attitudes are essential if you plan on coming back. During the introductory tour and orientation, take note of the staff as well as the StairMasters.

- Notice whether the facility is clean (check those showers) and well-ventilated, and that the premises, equipment, and workout areas are well-maintained. A gym that can't keep itself in good shape isn't likely to be able to help you.

- Ask yourself (honestly) whether there is a wide enough variety of classes to keep you interested. Are there enough instructors to go 'round? Enough equipment so you won't be kept waiting? (Visit at the same time of day or week you plan to be going, to find out.)

- Make sure the gym has the kind of members with whom you feel comfortable: Will being surrounded by muscle-bound Mr. and Ms. Universe types motivate you, or will they have you sobbing into your exercise towel as you sprint to the candy machine?

- Wear comfortable exercise clothing that doesn't leave you feeling overly exposed, and a good, lightweight set of headphones playing energizing music you really like. The more pleasant the *whole* experience, the fewer excuses you'll find to avoid it.

- Maximize your motivation: Arrange to meet a friend there. Make an appointment with a trainer. Leave something you need—and must return to get in a day or two—in your locker.

91

At least when it comes to alcoholic beverages. Bloody Marys, margaritas, piña coladas, and most every kind of daiquiri are just a few of the many mixed drinks that can be prepared sans liquor. Though for some of these drinks the caloric impact of the alcohol may not make a huge difference (the ingredients added to replace it can come close), eliminating the alcohol will help you resist many of the high-calorie drink accompaniments the liquor makes so hard to turn down. Or remember consuming.

92

Give your just-for-the-exercise walks a destination. Walking for the sake of walking is tedious, and the more tedious a task, the easier it is to talk yourself out of doing it. Set out with a specific goal—once around the neighborhood, to the post office and back, up and down every hallway on every floor in your apartment building— and you'll have the extra motivation of knowing your journey has a start *and* a finish.

93

 Give your just-for-the-exercise walks a deadline. Set a specific time to arrive at your goal and back, and you'll be less likely to dawdle. Want to walk a twenty-minute mile? Plan a one-mile course, and leave for it twenty minutes before a favorite television program begins. Want to walk faster tomorrow? Leave five minutes later.

94

 Establish baked-goods boundaries. Don't fall victim to the lure of bare-faced cakes or pies—undefined portion sizes are always the largest. Use decorative trim, a dot of icing, or a sliver of nut to indicate individual servings, and stick to one (or one-half) for yourself.

95

 Buy yourself a beautiful journal in which to write down everything you eat. And write it down! There's no better way to combat "food amnesia" and keep track of your calories. Promise to show or e-mail a copy of the journal entries to a supportive friend every week to keep you honest.

96

Ask a thin friend who eats well to write down what she eats for a week. We're not talking about those blessed creatures who stay skinny on a diet of chips and chocolates, but someone who has to maintain her weight consciously, and sensibly, like the rest of us mortals. Get a copy of her weekly menu (including serving sizes!), and follow it food for food, portion for portion.

97

Watch a skinny person eat and take note of his or her good habits. Then follow them.

98

TIP OF THE WEEK	KEEP A REWARD WISH LIST TO CELEBRATE YOUR ACCOMPLISHMENTS, AND MOTIVATE YOU TO MORE.

Some accomplishments are a reward in themselves: fitting into a dress you wore as a teenager, seeing your partner do a double take when he sees you in that new size 8. But for special milestones—either of reaching a goal (losing another ten pounds), or of doing what it takes to reach one (going a month without a chocolate binge)—a wish list of rewards (a.k.a. motivation) can help. Include pampering massages or facials, an appointment with the *best* hairstylist in town, or add extra slimming power to those milestones by listing wardrobe luxuries in that flattering color—a black cashmere sweater, black suede gloves, a black leather purse, black silk stockings, a sexy black nightgown.

99

When you check into a hotel, immediately relinquish the key to the mini-bar, and tell the hotel staff that you don't want it back. If your traveling companion complains, make him wear the key on a chain around his neck at all times, or hide it like another woman's phone number.

100

When you check into a hotel, turn in the contents of the mini-bar to the proper authorities, and replace them with healthy fruits, low-fat snacks, and beverages. Make sure you let the front desk know you didn't use the original contents—and that you don't want them replaced.

101

On vacation or business trips, find hotels with gyms on the premises, or that have arrangements with a local health club to allow their guests to visit for free. Some offer classes (sign up!) or fitness "room service," delivering exercise videos and equipment—from dumbbells to treadmills—to your door. A few will even arrange for a personal trainer. (If you belong to a gym, before taking an out-of-town trip ask whether it has visitors' privileges anywhere near your destination.) Use the gym at least once.

102

On vacation or business trips, walk the entire length and breadth of your hotel, motel, cruise ship—wherever you're staying. Every floor, every hallway, at least once every day. Not only will you get a good workout, but you'll get a better idea of whether you'll want to return in the future.

103

When you arrive at a hotel, don't ask where any of the facilities are located. Instead, take a walking expedition to find them. The longer you're lost, the more calories you'll burn.

104

Cut the calories when you bake by cutting the amount of extras in the recipe. Use half the chocolate chips in your cookie recipe; use half the walnuts in your brownies.

TIP OF THE WEEK	GO "HALFSIES."

Eliminating certain types of food from your diet "cold turkey" can be a wrenching experience that ends up backfiring; if you feel deprived and unhappy, you'll be more likely to eat even more of the stuff for revenge. There's a kinder, gentler alternative: Dilute those high-test products with lighter versions, and wean yourself as gradually as feels right for you.

LIGHTEN	BY BLENDING IT WITH
Ground red meat	Ground turkey, lower-fat vegetarian meat substitute, bread shreds, cracker crumbs
Ketchup	Salsa
Sugar	Low- or no-calorie sweetener
Salt	Light salt, then salt substitute
Cream	Half-and-half, then milk, then reduced-fat milk; or fat-free nondairy creamer
Coffee or tea	Decaffeinated coffee or tea
Stick butter or margarine	Light margarine, then light margarine in tubs (it's even lighter)

106

Build barricades. Securely seal any fattening food temptations (a.k.a. diet busters) in your household with multiple layers of plastic wrap and lots of tape to slow you down and allow you more time to resist their siren song. A layer or two of aluminum foil will provide extra armor. If you're really serious, go for the duct tape.

107

Establish a quarantine. Quarantine yourself against those nasty diet busters—whenever possible, don't allow them into your house. When you do your food shopping, avoid (like the plague) the aisles in which they're located, or whisk past those areas at the very end of the trip, when you've had it with food shopping and want to get out of the market.

108

When you throw food in the trash, thoroughly bury it under more trash so there will be absolutely no question of changing your mind, and "rescuing," say, a neatly discarded dessert later on.

109

Whether you're eating at home or in a restaurant, have your salad dressing served on the side, and dip your empty fork—not your veggies—into it before spearing a bite to eat. You'll cut way down on the amount of dressing you use.

110

Divide the food on your plate in half, and eat only what's on the right side. You'll halve the calories, and have leftovers for another meal. Package the left side before you're tempted to rotate the plate.

111

Sabotage the enemy. When an overloaded dinner or dessert plate is set before you, and you can't get the excess packed up or otherwise removed quickly enough, sabotage what you want to avoid overeating. Shake sugar onto the mashed potatoes, lace fish bones into the rice, pour pepper onto the layer cake or some water into the ice cream. Salt, ketchup, hot sauce, and ashes are other weapons of choice.

112

A beautiful environment discourages ugly eating: bingeing, pigging out, or trashing yourself with junk food. One caveat: The scent of the blooms can affect your appetite. While a light aroma may complement the dining experience, a heavy fragrance can leave you gagging. Set the table with stargazer lilies and hyacinth only if you want to skip the meal altogether.

113

Eat with your family, but don't gain weight with them. Just because the rest of the household isn't interested in losing weight doesn't mean you can't. Remember: The family that eats together doesn't have to eat the same thing.

114

Chew each mouthful at least twenty times. Not only is the digestion of smaller pieces of food easier on your gastrointestinal system, but the more slowly you eat, the less you'll consume before your brain gets the message that your stomach is full. (There's about a twenty-minute delay between the time your stomach reaches its satiation point and the time your head finds out about it.)

115

Use smaller utensils to slow you down, and give your brain more time to receive your stomach's "I'm full!" signal. You'll also feel like you're getting more food per bite.

116

Put down your knife and fork between bites to slow you down and give your brain more time to receive your stomach's "I'm full!" signal.

117

Get to work without rolling up your sleeves. Pushing or rolling up your sleeves is fine for getting down to work, but remember that the area of your arms to which you push or roll them will instantly gain a few inches. If you must, roll sleeves so that the hem forms not a widening horizontal, but a toward-the-body diagonal.

118

Don't let flared sleeves flare hips. When your arms are at your sides, the flare of a long sleeve falls at wrist level, and wrist level falls at hip level. You get the idea. Tapered sleeves are a better bet—not only will they spare your hips extra inches, but they allow some space to peek out between your arms and waist, and keep you from appearing to be one solid mass.

119

The more comfortable your feet feel, the happier they'll be to go on a nice, long, calorie-burning walk or run. Remember: Not all footwear is alike. A wide array is available to offer support of all kinds, appropriate for the stress exerted on different areas of the foot during different activities, from strolling to sprinting to aerobics to tennis. Start off with a good, basic cross-training shoe, and a good pair of insulating socks. Shop for them in the afternoon (when your feet have swelled slightly), at a specialized athletic shoe store with experienced fitters who'll do more than point you at a wall of boxes and wish you luck.

120

TIP OF THE MONTH   **HAVE EXTRA SALAD. ALL YOU WANT.**

Allow yourself something you can eat a whole lot of for those times when your hunger won't quit. Be sure, though, to take it easy on the dressing as well as the higher-carbohydrate and higher-fat toppings—just because something's served in a bowl with lettuce doesn't make it calorie- and fat-free.

LOAD UP ON	TAKE IT EASY ON
Lettuces and greens (especially nutritious dark-leaf varieties)	Dressing
	Shredded or diced cheese
	Croutons
Radish, cucumber, and zucchini rounds	Bacon bits (real or imitation)
	Olives
Colorful peppers (red, green, yellow, orange, purple)	Strips of luncheon meat
	Chickpeas (garbanzo beans)
Broccoli and cauliflower florets	Nuts and seeds
	Avocado
Carrot shreds	Hard-boiled egg
Asparagus spears	Pickled or marinated veggies
Sprouts	Oil
Tomatoes (plum, cherry, grape)	
Beets	
Hearts of palm	
Scallions and onions	
Mushrooms	
Capers	
Lemon	
Vinegar	

121

Use "thinkthin" as a computer password. Every time you log on you'll be reminded.

122

Buy better clothing. A penny saved is a pound you look like you've gained. Sizes really do run smaller in cheaper clothing, and that means finding something large enough to accommodate one part of your body can require buying a larger size than you'd otherwise need. The result: A garment that fits one area fine, and swims on you (read: makes you look heavier) elsewhere. Not worth it. And yuck.

123

If it's pleated, delete it. Pleated pants are great for anyone who actually *wants* a paunchier tummy—you don't even need to *have* a bulge for them to make it look as though you do. Pleated skirts stretch around your wider areas as if to emphasize them. Unless pleats lie so flat that they can barely be detected, forgo them.

124

Gather your gathered clothing and get rid of it. Can something also known as "bunching" be slimming? We think not.

125

Get your ice cream "fix" from the world's tiniest spoons. Why commit to a pint, or even a cone, when a sample-spoon-size taste at the local ice cream parlor will suffice? Embarrassed to taste and not buy? Try the White Rabbit Technique: Sample this, sample that, look at your watch, gasp loudly, and run. "I'm late! I'm late! So sorry! Gotta go!"

126

TIP OF THE WEEK	TAKE FIVE STEPS TO HAPPY HOUR HAPPINESS (OR, HOW TO HANDLE FREE FOOD AND HALF-PRICE LIQUOR WITHOUT DOUBLING YOUR WEIGHT).

Greasy ribs, fried wings, meatballs swimming in sauce, and platters of cheese are hard enough to resist. Serve them buffet-style, combine them with the inhibition-ridding power of two-for-one alcoholic beverages, and offer them for free, and it's a diet disaster in the making. A Happy Hour, maybe; an unhappy week on the scale for sure. But this does not mean you need to exclude yourself from one of America's great after-work pastimes. We say be thin *and* happy.

Step 1. Have a filling, low-calorie snack (a low-calorie nutrition bar, or a piece of fruit, for instance) before arriving at the restaurant or pub.

Step 2. Allow yourself one trip to the buffet table, and one plate to fill.

Step 3. Make that trip before you have had even one sip of an alcoholic beverage.

Step 4. After surveying the table, load your plate with any and all fresh fruits and vegetables in sight. Celery and carrot sticks, broccoli and cauliflower florets are often available, and you are allowed to snatch the cherry tomato garnishes from the cheese plate. Skip the heavy dip that's usually offered with the veggies, and ask a waiter to bring you a portion of low-calorie salad dressing when you get back to your seat.

Step 5. Take five. On the last bit of space remaining on your plate, squeeze up to five other small items of your choice: two wings and three ribs; one egg roll, one pig in a blanket, two ravioli squares, and a cube of cheddar. Follow with a big, healthy salad, and call it dinner.

127

If you like white wine, drink red wine. If you like red wine, drink white wine. If you like scotch, drink vodka. In other words, select something you're less likely to enjoy, and you'll drink less of it.

128

If you want half the calories, order half the drink. Even the most humble neighborhood tavern is equipped with an impressive array of glassware. Ask the bartender to use a smaller glass.

129

Pace your alcohol consumption. Take one sip for every four sips taken by your companion.

130

Drink it straight up. High-calorie alcoholic beverages go down very easily when the alcohol is hidden in fruit juice, sodas, cream, and the like. Skip the mixers and you'll be amazed at how much longer you hold the same glass. (Plus, you'll avoid the calories those mixers contain.)

131

 Buy expensive liquor. The higher the price tag, the slower you'll drink.

132

 Put big, bright, star-shaped stickers on the "good" foods in your kitchen. They'll attract your eye when you need to make a smart decision in a hurry.

133

TIP OF THE **WEEK**	**TAKE SNACKS ON THE ROAD.**

 No, not chips or chocolate bars, but healthy choices like dried veggies or fruits, so that you're not ravenous by the time you drive up to your kitchen door, your office, or even the restaurant or hotel you've been traveling so long to get to. Glove-box goodies are also a great defense against the temptation of any fast-food eateries whose drive-through windows beckon. Grab a handful of dried fruits or sun-dried tomatoes, a low-calorie snack bar, or a refreshing gulp of bottled water (freeze the water in advance and it will stay cold for hours), for willpower-to-go.

134

Allow yourself one sample of each "souvenir food" per vacation spot. Philadelphia is famous for its cheese steak, Maine for its lobster, New Orleans for jambalaya and beignets. You get the idea. Enjoy one full-fledged, can't-get-it-like-this-anywhere-else portion per visit, and you won't have to console yourself by overeating when you get home.

135

Park your car farther away from your destination, or get off the bus or train a stop early, and walk the extra distance. Any additional physical activity you can work into your day will burn off additional calories and pounds.

136

Give your bus or train seat to someone else, and stand. Standing burns more calories than sitting, especially when you're keeping your balance in a moving vehicle. If nobody else wants your seat, stand anyway.

137

Take the stairs instead of the elevator or escalator. If you must use the escalator, don't just stand there—walk along with it.

138

Bypass the automatic entries of stores and office buildings, and open those doors yourself for some quick resistance exercise. Extra credit if you hold the door open for others. (Unless they, too, want to consider it resistance exercise, and resist your offer.)

139

Fidget. Whether you're on the phone, in line at the bank, or in the waiting room at the dentist, stand up and start walking. Pace. Shift from one foot to the other. Burn extra calories and lose extra weight.

140

TIP OF THE WEEK	GO TO THE GARDEN.

Not only is it a safe distance from the kitchen, but the great outdoors is a great place to work off a lot of the calories you took from it, and your muscles will benefit in shapely ways. Digging and shoveling help tone legs, stomach, arms, and shoulders; stirring a compost heap with a spading fork strengthens arms, shoulders, and back; shearing the hedge will strengthen arms, shoulders, and chest.

- Use a push mower instead of a riding mower; better yet, use a push mower that isn't motorized. If your lawn is too big, do one section at a time.

- Mix it up. Alternate high-energy tasks like digging with easier chores like weeding or dead-heading flowers.

- Replace electric hedge clippers with hand-powered shears, and trim more lightly, and more often.

- Increase your range of motion or add weight resistance to a garden activity (swing the shovel more widely, pick up more soil at a time).

- Spend thirty calorie-burning minutes amongst the flora and fauna at least once a week. (You might even get a slimming tan.) Here are some typical results:

ACTIVITY	CALORIES
Mowing with a riding mower	101
Planting seedlings	162
Raking	162
Trimming shrubs	182
Weeding	182
Mowing with a motorized push mower	182
Laying sod	202
Chopping wood	243
Mowing with a push mower	243
Digging or shoveling	300

141

Leave your keys and umbrellas as far from the door as possible. Upstairs, in the basement, or simply on the other side of your home. Jog to get them. Jog to put them away.

142

If your vacation plans include an amusement park, call ahead or check the park's website to find the concession stands at which you'll be able to make the fewest concessions in terms of your diet.

143

When you fly, order a special meal in advance. Most airlines have menus to suit everyone from dieters and vegetarians to those who follow Kosher or Hindu dietary laws. One major domestic carrier offers fourteen choices (not counting three children's meals), including three vegetarian selections. And there's no extra charge. Call or check the airline's website to find out about your low-calorie options; you can usually request your preference up to two days before the flight.

144

When you fly, *look* at the airline food. Really closely. Need we say more?

145

Do "airport aerobics." Airports are filled with conveniences, from moving sidewalks to shuttles and trains that will transport you to your gate. Don't use any of them.

146

Want chocolate? Eat a sour pickle. The aftertaste will turn your sweet tooth into something else altogether. (Think of it as Antabuse for chocoholics.)

147

TIP OF THE WEEK   **PROCLAIM A FRUIT TUESDAY.**

Every now and then, dedicate the day to this deliciously colorful, mostly low-fat food group (sorry, avocado). Enjoy your old favorites, and try something new.

FRUIT	CALORIES/ CALORIES FROM FAT
Apple	80/0
Avocado, California, ⅕	55/45
Banana	110/0
Cantaloupe, ¼	50/0
Cherries, 1 cup	90/0
Grapefruit, ½	60/0
Grapes, 1½ cups	90/10
Honeydew melon, ¹⁄₁₀	50/0
Kiwifruit	50/5
Nectarine	70/0
Orange	70/0
Peach	40/0
Pear	100/10
Pineapple, ¾-inch-thick slice	30/0
Plum	40/5
Strawberries, 8	45/0
Tangerine	50/0
Watermelon, 2 cups	80/0

148

 Take your dog for a brisk walk. Good for you *and* your pup. Count his tree- or hydrant-sniffing as your warm-up, then hit the trail at a swifter pace. Cool down with another round of sniffing before returning home. If your dog is too small for "brisk," carry him. (If you have two small dogs, think hand weights.)

149

Take *your friend's dog* for a brisk walk. Make your friend come along. Good for you, your friend's dog, your friend, and your friendship. If she doesn't have a dog, take *her* for a walk.

150

Volunteer at the local animal shelter and walk *all* the dogs.

151

TIP OF THE MONTH

BRAVE THE BEACH.

Yes, you can wear a swimsuit, and look *good* in it.

- Take advantage of suits with built-in underwires, tummy panels, and high Lycra content to provide support.

- Stay away from shiny fabrics, which accentuate bulge.

- Close-fitting swimsuits in a print or pattern are more forgiving than solid-color suits. Choose a small, simple print, or well-placed stripes.

- Find a private dressing room with a multiview mirror and take in as many suits as you can carry, including larger sizes that won't cut into your flesh. No one is looking—try on *everything!*

- If you can't find a one-piece suit that suits you, try a tankini: a tank top and high-waisted bikini bottom that can often be purchased separately, in sizes to fit each part of you.

- Choose suits with high-cut legs to make yours look longer and thinner.

- Wear the right footwear. Flat flip-flops are fattening. Wear beach- and pool-friendly wedge sandals to make your legs look longer.

- Beach cover-ups cover a multitude of sins. Pass up the bulky cotton terry cloth in favor of long, flowing fabrics that complement your suit. Even a long gauzy shirt will do. Sarongs are another great way to hide everything you want hidden: Tie the soft expanses of fabric above the bust or on the hips (just don't pull too tight).

- And when all else fails, get into the water: It's *the* best cover-up, swimming in it is great exercise, and, with its lighter gravity, there's no quicker way to lose weight.

152

Get a tan. Tan looks thinner. Especially if you stand against tan backgrounds. Be sure to use adequate amounts of waterproof sunscreen—wrinkles and skin cancers are *not* attractive, no matter how slim you are.

153

Never say never. Run, do not walk, from all-or-nothing diets. Those that espouse a "never eat this" or "only eat that" philosophy are not only bad for your health, and ultimately doomed to failure, but they'll have you climbing the walls—and into the refrigerator and pantry—for exactly what it is that's prohibited. Don't leave any food "off your list," and you won't be as compelled to eat it.

154

TIP OF THE WEEK   **TAKE A FITNESS VACATION.**

No, not a vacation *from* fitness, but a vacation dedicated *to* it. Book a week or two at a spa, at a ranch, at a ski chalet—anyplace that involves movement other than that which takes place around the buffet table. Classic favorites:

- Bicycle tours

- Fall foliage hikes

- Dude ranches

- Birdwatching walks

- Diving expeditions

- Mountain climbs

But that's only the beginning. Discover the world of "adventure travel," where there's something for every interest, and at every level of physical activity, from archaeological digs to whale watching, from mountain biking in Mongolia to bungee jumping in New Zealand. You can even be a kid again, at summer sports camps of all kinds. See a travel agent or search the Internet for adventure tour operators, which specialize in different areas of interest and areas of the world.

Not only will you enjoy a great vacation, but you'll jump-start your metabolism—and your weight-loss mind-set—in a way that will last for weeks afterward. Note: Before you book any trip, double-check the level of activity involved, and find out what physical condition you're expected to be in.

155

Mail yourself a beautiful reminder. Treat yourself to a box of the prettiest note cards you can find. On each card, write one reason why the new, thinner you will be a happier, more beautiful you:

a you in better health, a you with more energy, a you who can slip into that gorgeous red dress you've been eyeing for months. (Photographs are allowed.) Seal each note in a stamped, self-addressed envelope, and give the whole box to a dependable friend with instructions to put one card in the mail every week.

156

Have friends mail you beautiful reminders. Treat yourself to a second box of beautiful note cards. Stamp and self-address all the envelopes, and date each one (at one-week intervals) in the lower left-hand corner. Give one card and envelope to each of your supportive friends or family members, with the request that they write a note of encouragement to you. Ask them to mail their notes on the date written on their envelope.

157

When you're invited to be a dinner guest, maintain your weight-loss integrity by offering to bring a delicious low-fat, low-calorie dish: a big, beautiful salad; a hearty, healthy casserole; a great fresh fruit dessert. No matter what's being served, you'll have a guilt-free option available.

158

Tighten your belt before you eat. We're not just talking in terms of your diet plan, but literally. Take it in a notch or two. Or wear a smaller belt. You'll be more conscious of your expanding waistline if your midsection feels the pinch.

159

Switch to "high octane" breath mints. Under the right circumstances, even Tic Tacs can trigger a binge. As low-calorie as they are, it's not the calories that are the concern, but the bingeing itself, which can start a cycle that can move into the higher-calorie food items with ease. Opt for refreshing sprays, drops, or mints like those we found in tins bearing the warning "hypercharged"—so strong that chewing even one proved a challenge. (Not to mention the physical exertion involved in opening the tin . . .)

160

Every time you're tempted to eat something fattening, picture the face (and body) of that thin friend who insists that you don't need to lose weight, and foists her desserts and her gift boxes of chocolates off on you. Remind your sweet tooth that *revenge* is sweet. Get back at her.

Every now and then, *you* mow the lawn, rake the leaves, and take out the garbage. Not only will you work off a wheelbarrow full of calories, but he'll owe you big-time. Here are the calories you might burn from thirty minutes of such kindness:

ACTIVITY	CALORIES
Mowing the lawn (riding mower)	101
Washing and waxing the car	150
Raking	162
Mowing (push mower with motor)	182
Blowing snow	200
Stacking firewood	200
Carrying a fifty-pound object	216
Chopping wood	243
Mowing (push mower)	243
Shoveling snow	300

162

Don't cook. More and more food services and gourmet markets are expanding their menus to satisfy dietary requirements of every kind, including those of the calorie-conscious. Whether you order an individual meal or cater the family's big holiday extravaganza, having someone else to do the cooking eliminates the risk of a meal's worth of premeal taste-testing.

163

Avoid large plaids. Unless you really *are* a lumber-jack, there's just no reason for this, or other large patterns. Stick with small prints of all kinds; best yet, small angular patterns on a dark field of color ("wear round" equals "look round").

164

Enrich your wardrobe with slimming colors. Consider them "the other blacks"—a spectrum of rich hues that can slim and flatter, especially when worn monochromatically. Like any good dark color, they are more figure-forgiving, they don't create shadows or shading around your rounder parts, and they can make even inexpensive garb look better made. Deep teal, burgundy, crimson, scarlet, violet, midnight blue, pine green, charcoal gray—all will work deliciously in your wardrobe palette. Rejoice: Here's one place where chocolate can make you *thin*.

165

Look at fabric patterns from a distance to check their direction. A material doesn't have to be covered with stripes to have a slimming vertical or nonflattering horizontal effect. To see where a pattern is going, step back about ten feet and narrow your eyes. The details will disappear and the direction will be revealed.

166

Leave furry and fuzzy to the stuffed animals. They look cute when they look chubby. You don't.

167

Serve your salad fixings "salad-bar style." Do it right, and your family will stop whining over their missing croutons and cheese cubes, while you can enjoy your salad without the guilt (about their suffering *or* about your consumption of fattening foods). In a large salad bowl, toss a super-low-calorie mix of greens, tomatoes, mushrooms, cucumbers, carrots, peppers, radishes, onions, and any other veggies with calorie counts almost too low to matter. Serve the more fattening garnishments—from avocado wedges to bacon bits—in individual ramekins or small bowls, as far from your own place setting as possible.

Every now and then dedicate the day to this deliciously colorful, low-fat food group. Enjoy your old favorites, and try something new.

VEGETABLE	CALORIES/ CALORIES FROM FAT
Asparagus spear	5/0
Bell pepper	30/0
Broccoli stalk	45/0
Carrot	35/0
Cauliflower, ⅙ head	25/0
Celery stalk	10/0
Cucumber, ⅓	15/0
Green (snap) beans, ¾ cup	25/0
Green cabbage, ¼ cup	25/0
Iceberg lettuce, ⅙ head	15/0
Leaf lettuce, 1/12 head	15/0
Mushroom	4/0
Onion	60/0
Potato	100/0
Radishes, 7	15/0
Summer squash, ½	20/0
Sweet corn	80/10
Sweet potato	130/0
Tomato	35/0
Winter squash, ½ cup	65/0

Note: The summer squashes, such as yellow crookneck and zucchini, have fewer calories than the winter squashes, such as acorn and butternut. How to remember which is which, and what will keep you leaner? Easy: Summer squashes are often longer and *thinner* in shape, and have *thin* skins; winter squashes are usually *rounder,* and their skins are *thick.*

169

Buy an enormous, gorgeous salad bowl and a great set of tongs to go with it. It will encourage you to fill it to the brim with equally gorgeous veggies. And to eat them!

170

Switch to a flavor or brand of food or drink you can more easily resist. Adore strawberry ice cream? Buy pistachio. Head over heels for Häagen-Dazs? Buy the supermarket brand.

171

When you arrive at a hotel, tell room service to mark your room as one that will *not* be served, no matter how hard you beg or plead. Tell man-agement you're willing to sign a sworn statement to the effect that your cries won't be loud enough to disturb other guests.

172

If you're staying at a hotel that serves a breakfast buffet, bring some fruit back to your room for pick-me-ups throughout the day, or to take along on day trips or tours. Gloat as your traveling companions pay the gastronomic consequences of roadside fare.

173

Carry your own luggage. Why should the bell-hops get all the good muscles?

174

On vacation, book yourself into every walking tour that is offered.

175

 Include anything from a jump rope or hand-weights, to a high-tech digital scale, to exercise clothing you're comfortable to be seen in as well as comfortable to work out in. (Stumped? Look for tips with symbols beside them.) Be specific and, most important, let your gift-givers know that you *have* a wish list and where you keep it. And remember: You *are* allowed to fulfill your own wishes!

176

 Don't sit longer than thirty minutes at a time. Take a five-minute break to get up, stretch, and do something on your feet.

177

 Jog to the corner mailbox and home again every time there's something to post. Mail one envelope at a time.

178

At restaurants, order a light appetizer or two side dishes as an entrée. Add a side salad to round out the meal.

179

Never order anything involving the words "deluxe," "super size," or "jumbo."

180

Order from the children's menu. You'll be served a smaller portion, and sometimes you even get a toy.

181

TIP OF THE MONTH

LEARN "MENUSPEAK."

The words used to describe the food on a menu can help you gauge the fat content of the meal.

LIGHTER FARE	HEAVIER FARE
Au jus	Alfredo
Au vin	Almondine
Baked (except cakes!)	Au gratin
Balsamic	Basted

LIGHTER FARE	HEAVIER FARE
Braised	Batter-dipped
Broiled	Béarnaise
Consommé	Béchamel
Dry rub	Beurre blanc
En brochette	Bordelaise
Fat-free	Breaded
Fresh	Buttery
Fruit glaze	Cheese
Fruit-sweetened	Creamed
Grilled	Crème fraîche
Herb-crusted	Crispy
Light	Croissant
Low-calorie	Crunchy
Low-fat	En casserole
Marinara	En croûte
Marinated	Filo wrapped
Oil-free	Fried
Poached	Gravy
Red sauce	Hollandaise
Reduction	Parmigiana
Roasted	Puff pastry
Seared	Rich
Steamed	Sautéed
Stir-fried in broth	Scalloped
Tomato-based	Smothered
Vegetable-based	Stir-fried in oil
Vinaigrette	Stuffed
Whole-grain	Tempura
Yogurt	

TIP OF THE WEEK	"CUT" YOUR SALT WITH LIGHT SALT OR DO WITHOUT IT ALTOGETHER.

Although the body needs about 500 milligrams of sodium (a.k.a. salt) a day, most of us consume at least eight times as much, and that without the salt shaker's help. Excess sodium causes your body to retain water, and can leave you feeling and looking bloated and heavy—not to mention the adverse effect on your blood pressure. Look out for a mine of salt in many foods, especially those that are canned (soups, vegetables), cured (bacon, ham), or otherwise processed (luncheon meats). Ketchup, mustard, soy sauce, baking powder, baking soda, and carbonated beverages are other culprits. Here, the sodium you'd find in 100 grams (3½ ounces) of some favorites:

FOOD	MILLIGRAMS OF SODIUM
Canned crabmeat	1,000
Frankfurter	1,100
Saltines	1,100
Bologna	1,300
Dill pickle	1,428
Pretzels	1,680
Corned beef	1,740
Parmesan cheese	1,862
Canadian bacon	2,500
Dried beef	4,300

183

Reduce or eliminate your caffeine intake. Caffeine, like salt, causes your body to retain water. And, like sugar, it will excite blood sugar levels and can prompt food cravings. Watch for it not just in coffee, but in tea, carbonated beverages, and, yes, chocolate.

184

Dress for success, holiday style. No loose pants or muumuus allowed—you want to remain conscious of the stomach expansion that so often takes place at (and around) the table. You also want to look *smashing* (which rules out the muumuu)! Tailored slacks or skirts, a comfortably cinched belt or sash, or an ever-so-slightly constrictive foundation garment will keep you aware of your waistline, and looking great. While you're at it, splurge on some fabulously expensive lipstick: You'll be less inclined to indulge in any unladylike gorging.

185

Dress in proportion. Combine longer blouses with shorter skirts, or shorter blouses with longer skirts, for a one-third/two-third proportion that will keep your body from looking like it's been divided in half.

186

Coordinate your belt color to your advantage. If you're short-waisted (the distance from your waist to your shoulders is less than the distance from your waist to the top of your thighs), match your belt to your blouse to extend the length of your torso. If you're long-waisted, match your belt to your slacks for the opposite effect.

187

Wear more where there's less of you. Distract eyes from the areas you have more of by putting the emphasis where you have less. If you're bottom heavy, try wearing small shoulder pads, pairing looser blouses with more tailored skirts or slacks, or otherwise dressing up your top. If you're top heavy, go easy on the necklaces, and wear lighter-weight blouses with as little detailing (buttons, pockets, decorative seams) as you can find.

188

Go easy on the layering. It adds layers to you.

Take a cool new approach to bananas and grapes, peaches and berries, and other fruits. Not only are they delicious frozen treats, but once they're chilled, they will take longer to eat than they would at room temperature. Remember to peel the banana *before* you wrap it in plastic or seal it in a zip-lock bag to freeze. Better yet, slice it into halves, quarters, or slices, so you can enjoy a tasty treat without having to eat (or resist) the whole fruit at once. Wrap and freeze the berries in batches of five or ten; do the same with the grapes, after removing them from the stem.

Most delicious: For a cornucopia of frozen delight, freeze fruit kabobs—skewers of sliced peaches, mangos, grapes, bananas, melon balls, even kiwis.

190

Freeze 'n' don't eat. Put candy bars and other sweet temptations into the freezer to slow you down when you get the urge. (A frozen Milky Way is delicious, but biting into one takes time and *care.*) Better yet, put them in the back of the freezer to help you resist the temptation further. You won't see them as easily, and if you have to take everything out to get to them, you'll have the chance to think twice about eating them at all.

191

Purge your refrigerator and pantry. Dispose of all the hidden-away-back-there temptations that seem to move to the front by themselves when you're most susceptible. Tempt a supportive friend to help you—and keep you from cleaning the contents into your open mouth—with the promise that she gets to keep all the food you toss. Work fast and hard—the more energetically it's done, the less temptation for you, and the more calories you'll burn in the process.

192

Buy a fat-women-in-bikinis calendar, and tape it to your refrigerator door. If your family protests that you're ruining everyone else's appetite in addition to your own, use a slightly more discreet, fat-woman-in-a-bikini postcard instead.

193

Buy a good full-length, front-, side-, and rear-view mirror so you can honestly see what all of you looks like, and how good success will look on you. It will also help you remember why you want to lose that weight to begin with, and encourage you to dress thinner along the way.

194

Cross your legs at your ankles. Not because you want to look like a good girl, but so your thighs and calves will look slimmer. And you'll have a better chance of getting to be a bad girl.

195

Take your diet to the movies. Movie theaters are renowned for some of the highest-fat and -calorie popcorn around (not to mention the Milk Duds and Raisinets). Smuggle in your own snacks: air-popped popcorn, a fresh fruit, some chewy dried fruits or veggies. Or order a "kid's movie meal" with diet soda and a smaller portion of popcorn.

196

TIP OF THE WEEK   GIVE WINGS TO YOUR DIET.

Leave the airline food on the ground. Pack a healthy, nonfattening meal you prepared yourself or picked up from a local gourmet shop. Be sure your selections don't need refrigeration to stay fresh during the wait before your meal (factor in flight delays); to be on the safe side, stow a small freezer pack in your carry-on bag. A light cold-cut or cheese sandwich, a hard-boiled egg, a zip-lock bag of fresh veggies with an individual serving of low-fat dressing, fresh or dried fruit, a snack-size yogurt, fat-free pretzels, nutrition bars—all travel well and will get you through most domestic flights. And don't forget the sugar-free gum, suckers, or candies. Then sit back, buckle up, and gloat amidst the covetous looks of fellow travelers stuck with airline food.

197

To stay hydrated and full during an airline flight, when the flight attendant approaches you with the beverage cart, ask for a few extra bottles of water before the cart vanishes for the rest of the trip. Caution: If you don't have an aisle seat, drink at your own risk.

198

Turn up the heat. Use hot sauce, Tabasco sauce, horseradish, spicy mustards, wasabi, and any kind of pepper (from crushed red to jalapeño) to heat up your food, and cool down the speed at which you eat it.

199

Grill. It's not just for hot dogs and hamburgers. A wide variety of food can be prepared on the grill with less fat and fewer calories than most oven-cooked meals. Choose lean cuts of meat or, better, chicken, seafood, or veggies. Neither do the grill-food accompaniments need to be fattening: Replace the ketchup with salsa or other condiments (see Tip 329), replace the fries with grilled veggies and corn on the cob (use a little diet salad dressing to add flavor), replace the Bud with Bud Light, and serve with the biggest, most colorful salad you can toss.

200

Keep your hem away from your calf. Skirts or cropped pants will widen the part of the leg at which they are hemmed, so if you have heavy calves, aim slightly below them.

201

Let overblouses flow past your stomach and hips. Don't let the hem land a horizontal line across your widest areas. Blouses that fall just to the top of the thigh look better. Shirttail blouses, which lead the eye downward instead of across— and spare you extra fabric on the hips—look best.

202

Don't even *think* about hip-huggers. The lower your waistline, the shorter your legs look; and a hip-level horizontal line will make your widest part even wider looking. Not enough? Two words: bare stomach.

203

Too small, and you're liable to resemble two linked sausages—your tummy bulging over *and* under the constricting band. Too large, and you'll be wearing a look-at-my-hips hip-hugger. Test for fit in slacks and skirts by seeing whether you can easily slip your two thumbs inside the band without holding your breath. Next, hold that breath as deeply as possible, and use your thumb and forefinger to pinch the waistband fabric that remains. You should have no less than one inch of fabric, and no more than two between your fingers. (The "pinch test" can also be used for dresses.)

204

When you travel, reserve a hotel room on the highest floor possible, and use the stairs to get to and from it.

205

Reserve a hotel room as far from the lobby as possible. Not only will you get more exercise on the way to and from your quarters, but you'll think twice about visiting the lobby sweet shop.

206

To avoid temptations in hotel or motel snack-vending machines, bring along a small, can't-be-opened-without-a-hammer piggy bank, and empty all your change and small bills into it whenever you return to the room. Consider the savings a humble start toward your next vacation. Label the piggy bank "Next Vacation" or "Slinky Cruise-wear Ensemble."

207

Do it the hard way. For a calorie-burning boost, boycott convenience, be it the dishwasher, the riding lawnmower, the electric can opener, even the prewashed, precut veggies. Don't use the automatic garage-door opener either—get out and heft it yourself.

208

Share a restaurant order with your dining companion and split the calories.

209

Take cover under summer shawls and scarves. When it's too hot to wear anything that covers anything sufficiently enough, drape a lightweight, flowing expanse of gorgeous fabric over your shoulders to create a cool, long vertical line and cover a multitude of skin.

210

TIP OF THE WEEK	DO A HOUSEWORK WORKOUT.

Too much to do around the house to take time out for exercise? Wrong. You can exercise your rights to a clean home and a fit body at the very same time. Here's a list of some common activities, and the number of calories a 150-pound woman would burn by doing them for fifteen minutes:

ACTIVITY	CALORIES	ACTIVITY	CALORIES
Laundry	36	Vacuuming	68
Ironing	38	Washing windows	75
Washing dishes	41	Heavy cleaning	77
Light cleaning	43	Scrubbing the floor	99
Sweeping	45	Moving furniture	108
Making the bed	65		

211

Do a dishwasher workout. For an aerobic mini-workout, unload the dishwasher one item at a time, moving back and forth across your kitchen as energetically as you can without breaking dishes. For some weight-training practice, unload the machine in one fell swoop, stacking as many dishes as you safely can and lifting the whole pile at once.

TIP OF THE MONTH

212

RELAX.

Stress eating is not all in your mind. Hungry researchers report that even everyday nerve provokers, from ringing phones to screaming kids, can prompt the body to produce the stress hormone cortisol, which boosts appetite—especially appetite for carbohydrates and fat, which can whet the appetite further still. The more you stress, the more you eat, the more you stress. The good news: Once you learn to recognize that stress is the problem, you can calm it. Phew.

FIVE WAYS TO RECOGNIZE STRESS

Physical changes: such as rapid, shallow breathing; a pounding heartbeat, sweating, or trembling.

Emotional changes: including a shortened temper, or depression.

Mental changes: including absentmindedness, forgetfulness.

Sleeping pattern changes: whether more, less, or when.

Dietary changes: from what you feel like eating to how much of it you consume.

FIVE WAYS TO RELIEVE STRESS

Take a deep breath: Better yet, take several. It's called diaphragmatic breathing, and it really does work. Inhale through your nose on a slow count of five; then exhale through your mouth on a slow count of five. (Try thinking of the words "so" as you inhale, and "hum" as you exhale, and feel the difference.) If your stomach rather than your chest is moving, you're doing it right.

Move: Get physical. Take a walk; play some tennis; put on some lively music, and dance around your living room. Exercise is one of the most powerful stress busters there is, but stressing out about exercising is not. Have fun.

Get some sleep: When we need it most, it can be hardest to come by. Establish a bedtime routine to relax your body to slumber: a soothing bath, some stretches, a chapter of a relaxing book (no suspense thrillers allowed). And if you're up for a little under-the-covers activity before the snoozing sets in, all the better: The hormones and endorphins triggered by lovemaking cause the entire body to relax. Doctors' orders.

Laugh: It really can be the best medicine. Start a collection of favorite comic strips to look through.

Go out to see a comedy at the movies, or rent one from the local video store.

Schedule some quiet time: Block out a few hours for an appointment with yourself. Turn off the phones, extract yourself from your e-mail, turn on some relaxing music, or commune with Mother Nature.

213

Keep lapels long and narrow. So you will look that way too.

214

Don't belt jackets. The fabric on even the lightest jacket is bulky enough. Belting it just adds bunch.

215

Dress in a dress. There's nothing like it for a flattering, flowing, unbroken line from neck to hem. Choose tailored styles, nipped in slightly at the waist, with the hem slightly wider than the hips. With the right fabric and pattern, you'll achieve the ultimate vertical slimming effect.

216

Fill the need instead of feeding the need. Think about why you're eating: Is it hunger, or is it to take a work break? ("I'll finish this report as soon as I finish this doughnut.") Is it hunger, or is it to stay awake? ("Some cake and coffee will help me make it to the end of the late movie.") Find other things to do (take a walk to the office watercooler, videotape the movie and watch the end tomorrow) to fill the need.

217

TIP OF THE WEEK	CHOOSE HARD-TO-EAT FRUITS.

They're low in calories, high in taste, the seeds and peels will slow you down, and you can even claim some calorie-burning benefits from the physical exertion involved in opening them. Our favorites: oranges, tangerines, and clementines; grapefruits, papayas, mangos, and kiwifruits. For more exotic fare, try lychees, muscadines, passion fruit, pomegranates, sapodillas, and star fruit. And buy your grapes *with* seeds.

218

Drink a tall glass of water before every meal. It's a healthy way to quench your hunger. During-the-meal sips will fill you up even more.

219

Dive into water alternatives. You know water is good for your diet—and for you—but if that doesn't make it easier to swallow, try sparkling or mineral waters, or flavoring a glass with a splash of lemon or lime juice, a wedge of fruit, and some calorie-free sweetener. Alternatively, imbibe your water the hard way: chew ice.

220

Find a great hairstylist. The right one will help you find not the current fashion cut, but the right cut for *you*—for the shape of *your* face, the texture of *your* hair, the time *you're* prepared to put in every day to style it on your own. Tell her what you want, and listen to her suggestions before scissors touch hair. Consider visiting a few salons before deciding, and don't feel compelled to stay with a stylist who lets you down.

221

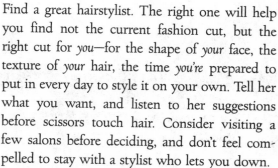

Keep a glass in your hand at parties to keep yourself occupied with something other than hors d'oeuvres. If you choose to make it an alcoholic beverage, alternate with a nonalcoholic diet soda or tonic to keep your willpower from washing away.

222

Replace your martini with a Gibson. For fewer calories and less fat, replace the martini's green olive with the Gibson's less-fattening pearl onion. Shake or stir.

223

Keep a beautiful journal of the compliments you get as you lose weight, and read them often.

224

TIP OF THE WEEK	WHEN YOU TRAVEL, PACK A PORTABLE GYM FOR A HEALTH-CLUB-TO-GO.

You can even get a mini-workout by packing it. Include:

- *One or two good exercise videos:* Stick to those led by a certified personal trainer who acknowledges the need for you to exercise at your own pace—and to rest.

- *A lightweight jump rope:* Choose a rope with nonslip foam grips. You'll know you have the right length if, when you step one foot on the center of the rope and bring both handles upward, the handles reach about chest high.

- *Portable free weights:* No need to tote heavy dumbbells in your luggage; special collapsible hand weights can be filled with water when you arrive.

- *Resistance tubes, loops, and bands:* Also known as exercise bands or, as a group, "lightweight rubber-resistive products," these light, stretchy, and very portable pieces of equipment can simulate loads from one to a thousand pounds of pressure when used in combination.

- *Comfortable exercise clothing:* Don't forget a good pair of aerobic or cross-training shoes, and socks.

225

When you sit at a bar, allocate a small portion of chips, pretzels, or other bar snacks to a cocktail napkin, break them into small pieces, and eat one at a time. Promise the bartender an extra nice tip if he'll take—and keep—the rest of the snacks away from you.

226

When you sit at a bar, promise the bartender an extra nice tip if he'll take—and keep—the snack foods away from you before you take any at all.

227

Don't sit at the bar.

228

Eat dessert only at restaurants, where it's served in individual portions and in public.

229

Keep your hands busy while you watch TV. They say idle hands are the devil's workshop. We say idle hands are the ones that are more likely to put food in your mouth. And when those idle hands are situated in front of the television, the likelihood increases exponentially, as you're assaulted with a regularly scheduled barrage of mouth-watering commercial messages. Keep those hands occupied: Do some needlework, doodle on a sketch pad, do your nails, give your partner a massage. Better yet, have him give you one.

230

Eat your "TV snacks" out of a bowl, not a bag. When you've "just gotta have it," prevent over-eating by limiting foods to a personal portion instead of taking the "I'll just grab a handful" approach. Low-calorie, low-fat, air-popped pop-corn is great for filling you up without filling you out—and there's enough in one portion to last through most sitcoms.

231

 Just because you don't see the word "sugar" on a food label doesn't mean it isn't there. If any of the following is first or second on the ingredients list, or several appear, watch out:

Corn sweetener	Lactose
Dextrose	Maltose
Fructose	Molasses
Fruit juice concentrate	Sucrose
Glucose	Sugar
Honey	Syrup

232

 Halve your recipes. If you prepare half as much, you'll eat half as much.

233

Buy a set of mini-muffin tins. With muffins that are half the size, you can enjoy two "eating occasions" for the calories and fat otherwise contained in just one.

234

Buy small salt-dip cups to use for individual salad dressing portions. If you can't find salt dips, egg cups will do.

235

Buy a colorful set of ramekins for snack portion control. Eat only as many chips or pretzels as will fit into one.

236

Use smaller dishes to reduce automatically the amount of food you can pile on. Dessert or salad plates can substitute for dinner plates all around the table—you'll serve less and it will look like more. If anyone asks, call it *tapas*.

237

Never eat out of a container. Don't tell *us* you have enough control not to empty the entire contents into your mouth. Make sure all your food has touched a plate.

238

On your next trip to the supermarket, find a product that weighs as much as the weight you've lost, grab it off the shelf, and tote it up and down the aisle a few times. You'll be amazed to realize how much excess baggage your body used to carry around, and you can better appreciate (and celebrate!) the fact that you've succeeded in casting it off. Progress from sticks of butter, to packaged meat, to bags of sugar, to sacks of kitty litter. "Just" five or ten pounds can feel a lot more significant when you're holding it in your hand.

239

Acknowledge that you're worth it. Consider the higher prices you often have to pay for individual portions and lower-fat foods at the supermarket to be a testament to your self-worth. "How bad do you really want to be thin?" they challenge us. "Enough to pay the extra cost?" Think of it this way: If you could hand someone the additional dollar and be guaranteed to lose weight, you'd do it in a second. And then you'd hand her another dollar. Think of this in the same way. You're worth the investment.

240

Schedule a personal photo session, or a family portrait, for motivation. Take one every other month, and watch as you take up less and less of the frame.

241

Trash the elastic. The only thing elastic waist-bands do is allow you to wear clothing far beyond the point at which you should have discarded it. Plus, they allow you to continue to expand.

242

Give your undergarments the Red-Line Test. If it takes more than ten minutes for the traces of your bra, panties, panty hose, or (confess) knee-highs to fade from your body, they're the kind of undergarments that will cause a bulge. Trade them in for the right size and fit.

TIP OF THE MONTH

ESTABLISH A FIRM, SLIM FOUNDATION.

Welcome to the twenty-first century, where new foundation fabrics and design have made it possible to look slimmer and keep breathing at the same time. These are not your mother's bras and girdles. They're comfortable, pretty, *and* effective. And at holiday dinners, the more constrictive variety of undergarments can help you from taking that second helping.

- For the torso, iron-maiden-style corsets have given way to a wondrous array of waist cinchers, bodysuits, body slips, tummy-toner panties, and derriere slimmers (and lifters!). Experience the softer, sexier fabrics, and you might not want to keep this underwear under wraps.

- Panty hose can do more than give you slimmer, shapelier legs. Try support hose, control top, and other styles designed to slim everything from waist to tummy to thighs.

- Underwire bras, minimizer bras, bras with side support, bustiers, front-closure bras, padded bras, push-up bras, convertible bras, sports bras, cami bras, demi bras, bandeaus . . . If you can't find one that will better your bustline, you just haven't looked. Stock up on a variety of bras appropriate for every outfit: seamless cups under a fine knit, sexy plunges for cleavage.

244

Vanquish VPL (Visible Panty Line). Where there's a line, there's a bulge. And where there's a bulge, there's an excuse to drown your sorrows in ice cream. Opt for panty-and-hose combinations, footless hose with tummy support, thong panties, or hold off until you better fit into those pants or skirts.

245

TIP OF THE WEEK	EAT LIKE A GROWN-UP.

Handfuls of cookies washed down with chocolate milk don't become anyone past age ten. When the kids get home from school, have a snack of your own prepared to help you resist the urge to join in eating theirs. As for your children's eating habits, cultivate their appreciation for healthier delights early on: Natural apple sauce, fresh or dried fruits, and frozen low-fat yogurt are a few possibilities that prove processed sugars aren't the only sweet treats.

246

Make a commitment to attend your high school or college reunion. Just as inviting guests to visit can compel you to clean house, a clear deadline and purpose will motivate you to shed extra pounds. No reunion? Make a date with an old classmate you want to impress.

247

Give one to the garden. For every dollar you spend on a fattening food, spend one dollar on a plant or shrub. Then get out in your garden and burn some calories planting it.

248

Go to sleep earlier, wake up later. At least take more naps. Yes, activity burns far more calories, but at least you won't be eating while you snooze.

249

Get rid of your "fat clothes" as you grow out of them. Don't allow yourself to fit back in. Consignment shops, charities, and fatter friends will be grateful. Too good to toss? Have your oversized apparel taken in by a tailor to flatter your new, slimmer figure.

250

Before you take a car trip, invest in a set of high-quality coolers and thermal packs in a variety of sizes to take on the road. Filled with healthy savories, they'll protect you from highway fast-food fatteners.

251

Bookmark your own fast food. Bookmark your favorite, fastest recipes in all your eating-light cookbooks. Keep the ingredients for at least three of them on hand, and you can have your meal ready before hunger allows that "other" fast food into your mouth.

252

TIP OF THE WEEK	DEVELOP A FIVE-MINUTE AT-WORK EXERCISE ROUTINE, AND DO IT TWICE A DAY.

They won't bring on a sweat and ruin your business attire, yet these simple repetitive motions can strengthen and tone muscles. Try any five of these for one minute each:

Desk pushaways: Stand two to three feet from your desk and place your hands flat on one of its edges (your body should be at a forty-five-degree angle from the floor, with your arms held straight).

Bending at the elbows, lower yourself toward the desk for a count of three, then straighten your arms for a count of three. Repeat.

File lifts: Pick up a box of file folders, ten filled file folders, or five "loaded" folders, and slowly lift them above your head. Slowly lower to waist level. Repeat. (If no file folders are available, a ream of bond paper will do just as well.)

Drawer pulls: While seated on your desk chair, grasp the handle of a drawer to your right and pull it open as far as it will go. Close the drawer. Repeat ten times. Now do the same with a drawer to your left.

Watercooler runs: Walk to the watercooler as quickly as you can, and then back to your office. Extra credit if you take the stairs to a watercooler on another floor.

Receiver lifts: Pick up the receiver of your telephone and hold it at arm's length, shoulder high. Bend at the elbow to bring the receiver to your ear and then away. Repeat with the other arm.

Chair rolls: Planting your feet on the floor, roll your chair slowly backward, then slowly forward, five times. Now try doing it to the sides.

Chair swivels: Planting your feet on the floor, slowly swivel side to side as far as you can.

Stapler clenches: Empty your stapler of staples, then, holding the device at arm's length, "staple" for counts of twenty. Use your right hand, then your left, holding your arm straight forward, straight out to the side, and then behind you.

Bookshelf rocks: Stand facing a bookshelf, with your feet two to three feet apart, and push off onto the ball of one foot and then the other so you rock from side to side. Why face a bookshelf? So your coworkers think you're working.

Staff meeting secrets: Pretend you're driving home, and try some "traffic-light isometrics" (see Tip 34) while the boss pontificates: Strengthen and tone your stomach or buttock muscles by clenching and then relaxing them. "Write the alphabet" (rotate your foot to "write" each letter), or do a few heel lifts (press down on the toes for a few seconds while lifting the heel) to shape calves. At least *something* productive will come out of the meeting.

253

Don't buy nuts without shells. Not only will the shells slow you down, but breaking into some practically qualifies as exercise. (We say, if you have the tenacity to break into a Brazil or coconut, you've earned it.)

254

Work for your snacks. Before you eat a high-calorie snack, clean the bathroom or vacuum the house. Don't eat until the faucets and sink are gleaming, or all the dust bunnies are gone.

255

Play for your snacks. Before you eat a high-calorie snack, work on a jigsaw, do a crossword puzzle, play a set of tennis. Don't eat until you place twenty-five pieces, fill in every across and every down, or win.

256

Don't give "insta-fat" a chance. You've seen it, you've felt it: the astonishing amount of weight gained in an instant over the holidays or on vacation. The bad news: The numbers on the scale can be discouraging enough to send you straight to the Sara Lee. The good news: If you attack before it "sticks" by getting right back on your diet, insta-fat will vanish as swiftly as it came.

257

Bench press a baby. No reason why weights have to be inanimate objects, and, done right (and safely), your little one will think you're a better ride than Magic Mountain. If you don't have your own, bench press a friend's baby. (And earn extra calorie-burning credits for sticking around to change his diaper.)

258

Skip dessert today.

259

TIP OF THE WEEK	HAVE A GOOD BREAKFAST.

The adage "Breakfast like a king, lunch like a prince, and dinner like a pauper" is good advice where weight loss is concerned. By getting a healthy start, you provide your body with the fuel it needs for the day ahead, and you'll be more likely to burn off that fuel instead of storing it as fat. (Every 3,500 calories you don't use are stored as one pound of fat. Use them or you *won't* lose them.) A substantial breakfast can also rev up your metabolism—temporarily boosting it by 10 percent or more.

We're not, however, talking about sugar-frosted flakes. Try a fruit or juice for natural sweetness;

a hearty bowl of whole-grain cereal, or a slice of toast, to round off your carbohydrates; light cottage cheese or even a dab of peanut butter for protein; and yogurt or skim milk for calcium. Just keep your low-fat, low-calorie interests in mind.

260

Get your calcium from something other than the cow. Eating enough dairy products to provide enough calcium for health can load on the fat grams. Spinach, broccoli, and calcium-fortified orange juice and cereals tend to be lower in fat and higher in other nutrients. Calorie-free calcium supplements are another good idea.

261

Opt for whole grains. They take the body longer to digest, so you'll feel full longer than you would if you ate other carbohydrates (which make blood sugar levels soar and plummet, and trigger hunger). Fill up on whole-wheat breads or pastas, beans, brown rice, or oats. The coarser ground, or closer to intact, the grain, the better.

262

Instead of cutting your bagel lengthwise in half, cut it in thirds. Give the center slice to a hungry friend, the trash can, or the birds.

263

Beware alcohol's "magnet" calories. It won't take much to convince yourself that spirits are relatively low in calories, and they are, after all, fat free. But remember that alcohol can attract additional calories to the ones in the glass by increasing your desire for and lowering your resistance to other foods—from the Beer Nuts on the bar to the brownies waiting for you at home. If "just say no" is hard when you're sober, intoxication will make it all the more difficult.

264

Eat before you drink that cocktail. Choose correctly, and the number of calories you'll consume in the form of the right foods is nothing compared to the calories in and "attracted to" your glass (see Tip 263). Even a modest amount of nourishment can slow intoxication's inhibition-ridding effects.

265

Avoid frozen alcoholic drinks. Not only are they bigger, and easier to down, but they tend to contain larger quantities of sugar than their straight or on-the-rocks counterparts.

266

BEWARE BAR FOOD.

What's beer without Beer Nuts? Wine without cheese? Most of the time, alcohol is not served alone, but with an arsenal of chips, pretzels, dips, crackers, nuts, and other assorted high-fat snacks. Choose wisely to minimize the damage.

FOOD	CALORIES/GRAMS OF FAT
Pretzel sticks, 10	10/0
Cheddar, 1-inch cube	70/6
Goldfish crackers, 60	75/3
Potato chips, 10	105/7
Snack mix, half cup	150/6
Peanuts, in the shell, 35	161/14
Peanuts, oil roasted, 35	165/14
Beer Nuts (cashew), 35	170/13
Beer Nuts (peanut, almond), 35	170/14
Mixed nuts with peanuts, 35	175/16
Macadamia nuts, 35	200/21

267

Visit the chat rooms of a reputable diet-oriented website for recipe ideas and encouragement. Many also provide interactive programs that allow you to compute the calories you'll burn for a wide range of activities, based on your weight and the time spent active. Do remember that some Internet entities are more reputable than others (aim for those ending in .edu, .gov, or .org), and that advice you get from a layperson is exactly that.

268

Start a light-cooking club. Find a like-minded friend or two for weekly experimentation. Together, shop for the ingredients, cook, and try out a new light meal, from salad to entrée to dessert. Celebrate your successes together.

269

Join an organized weight-loss group. Find one that takes a sensible approach, emphasizing a balanced eating program you can live with long term, a healthy amount of physical activity, and group support. Make sure meetings are easy to get to, so you have no excuse not to go. If multiple-meeting discounts are offered, sign up—acknowledge that one meeting alone won't do it, and make a long-term commitment to success.

270

 Don't wear white. It makes you look wider.

271

 Build an answer box. You know what challenges you most when you're trying to lose weight. (Your office's catered lunch meetings? The Girl Scout cookies your daughter brought home to sell?) You also know that when those challenges come, the answers to them are the last thing you remember. Be prepared: On individual index cards, write out what threatens you most and what helps you best. File them here, by category, so you can find them in a hurry.

272

 Act like a kid. Forget the formal exercise routine—run, jump, play around, and have fun!

273

| TIP OF THE WEEK | BRING YOUR INNER CHILD TO THE TABLE. |

 We highly recommend you confine the use of the following suggestions to the privacy of your own home.

Play with your food: Have fun with your food when nobody's looking, and make it last. Peel yourself a grape, suck out the center of a heart of palm, eat a sandwich crust-first.

Take the Oreo challenge: Nabisco says that the filling used in one year's production of these cookies could ice all the wedding cakes served in the United States for two years. So take your time. Split it, lick it, nibble around the edge. Go for the record. (Extra credit for using reduced-fat Oreos.)

Eat without utensils: This can really put a crimp in your mashed potato intake. (It also helps if you bring out your inner barbarian.)

Make your food funny: Take time to arrange it into the shape of a face, an animal, an hourglass figure.

Dawdle: Push your food around the plate. Sneak some to the dog. Count out one serving of reduced-sodium Goldfish crackers (sixty fishies!), and eat one per minute for an hour.

Fidget: Have you ever seen a child sit still at the table? Neither have we. Nothing burns calories like constant motion. Rock back and forth, pump your feet up and down, move, move, move!

BE AN INTERNATIONAL SUCCESS.

Know how to eat ethnic and the world is your oyster. We take that back; it's better than an oyster—it's a spring roll, and pasta, and fajitas.

CHINESE

Good news for dieters: Like many other types of Asian cuisine, the Chinese menu offers many lower-fat poultry, seafood, vegetable, and noodle dishes; is more likely to stir-fry than deep fry; and doesn't have a word for cheese.

Don'ts: Batter-dipped sweet and sour pork; anything involving the word "crispy"; egg rolls in fried wrappers (opt for vegetarian spring rolls, if you must); and nut-riddled, sauce-heavy dishes. Avoid fried rice in favor of steamed white or brown rice, or lighten its impact by mixing fried and steamed. And remember: Stir-fried foods, although better than deep-fried foods, are still . . . fried foods.

Do's: Opt for steamed or braised selections. Eat your Chinese food Chinese-style: Order a bowl of steamed white or brown rice and, instead of drowning the rice in any sauce your dish contains, use chopsticks (a.k.a. food brakes) to bring the food to the rice, one morsel at a time. Request reduced-sodium soy sauce, a limit on the nuts included in your dish, and more vegetables than meat in your meal. An order of steamed vegetables is a good accompaniment; the more you fill up on rice and steamed veggies, the less fat you'll consume, and the less likely you'll be hungry a half hour later.

ITALIAN

The Mediterranean diet goes easy on meat offerings and is renowned for its beneficial health effects—not the least of which is a lower risk of obesity. But that doesn't happen automatically when you walk inside the local *trattoria*.

Don'ts: Parmigiana anything; Alfredo anything; other buttery, cream-based, or cheese sauces; garlic bread; heavy red-meat and veal dishes; and pizza loaded down with cheeses and meats—especially fatty sausage, bacon, and pepperoni. Northern Italian food, renowned for its heavy-handed use of cheese, and cream sauces, is the greater challenge.

Do's: Southern Italian dishes favoring vegetable, sea-food, or chicken dishes; meatless, tomato-based marinara sauces, or (slightly higher in fat) pesto and tomato sauces. And, yes, pasta. If your entrée doesn't come with a side dish of pasta, order one and share it with your companions; like the rice in Chinese restaurants, it will help cut fat, and keep you full. A small slice of bread also helps—except for that slab of garlic bread slathered with butter and cheese. If you must, dip plain bread in a little olive oil, and sprinkle it with a pinch of Parmesan.

MEXICAN

You know a type of restaurant is dangerous when one of the most popular side dishes is beans that aren't just fried, but *refried*. Even Mexican rice is sautéed, and supercharged with calories and fat.

Don'ts: Beef- or cheese-stuffed anything; dishes cooked in oil (enchiladas), deep-fried (hard tacos), or immersed in boiling oil, filling and all (chimichangas); and the infamous cheese-filled, batter-dipped, deep-fried chile relleno. General rule: If it crunches, it's been fried. Stay away.

Do's: Fajitas, fajitas, fajitas—especially the vegetable, seafood, or chicken variety, as long as you don't go *loco* on toppings of the fat-loading kind: guacamole, sautéed onions, and sour cream topping the list. Other do's, with the same watch-the-toppings caveat: burritos, soft quesadillas, and soft tacos. Ask for beans that are *not* refried or, better yet, order à la carte and avoid both them and the rice altogether. Push the basket of tortilla chips to the other side of the table, or ask the waiter to remove them after you set aside a handful, and keep the flavorful yet fat-free salsa or pico de gallo nearby.

275

Tell if it's tight, and if so, toss it. Wearing something smaller than it should be will make you look larger than you are. Look for these telltale signs:

Cheshire crotch (that horrid grinning shape formed by pant creases)

Bunching, riding, or creeping

Horizontal creasing

Gaping buttons, or those that won't close

Stretched seams

Lasting impressions (of the clothing on your body when you take it off)

VPL or VBL (Visible Panty or Bra Line)

HBVP (Horizontal Bustline Valley Phenomenon)

Broken zippers or other fasteners

Ripping or shredding sounds

276

Use salsa instead of ketchup. It might not be taste alone that's made it the nation's number one condiment: salsa has only five calories per tablespoon (with one-half gram of sugars) versus ketchup's fifteen (with four grams of sugars).

277

Use scarves to draw eyes to your face and add a slimming vertical effect. Buy the most luxurious fabrics you can find, matching the weight of the scarf to the weight of your outfit. Play with a variety of shapes, ties, knots, loops, and draping styles to find the most flattering, and don't be afraid to ask a salesperson for help. In general, the shorter your neck, the narrower your scarf should be (fold it lengthwise if the cut is too broad). Just (a) don't disappear into it, and (b) avoid neck-shortening bandana styles.

278

Let necklines plunge, not boat. With the right cut, necklines are a beautiful way to draw attention to your face. Plunging necklines create a flattering vertical that not only elongates your neck but leads the eye in our favorite slimming direction. Boat necks and other horizontal styles create a wide horizon. You get the idea.

279

Avoid "bookshelf chest." Don't wear pendants long enough to rest on a well-endowed bust or dangle from it.

280

Having a short, specific period of time for physical activity makes it easier for even the exercise-challenged to tolerate. Keep a set of hand weights handy, and do a set of curls; push yourself up from the sofa for some push-ups or stretches; if your living room is spacious enough, you can even jump rope. Get up and *move* something until the sponsor has had his word—just keep that movement directed away from the fridge.

Other good exercise time frames: the time you wait for water to boil, the time you're on hold on the telephone, the time it takes for one cycle of the washing machine to complete.

281

Get your teeth professionally cleaned and whitened. You won't want to sully that gorgeous mouth with "bad" food.

282

Turn up the volume. Read the labels, and make the right choices to get more food for the same calories and fat. Foods don't even have to be marked "-substitute," "low calorie," or "low fat" to make a difference—try different brands or formulations, and be surprised.

283

Turn down the volume. Eat less of the substitute than would equal the original food to consume even fewer calories, and less fat. Buy your snacks in bite-size versions so you can still feel you're eating "the whole thing," and then eat fewer of them. (Five York Peppermint Pattie Bites, for instance, have the same number of calories as, and less fat than, one "snack size" Peppermint Pattie. Eat four Bites, or three Bites . . .)

284

Buy and use a step counter to see how many footsteps you take per day. It's a great way to gauge your activity, and the numbers add up much faster than if you were counting miles. Aim for five thousand, then six thousand, and so on.

285

Instead of driving to the store for a single bag of groceries, take a knapsack, and walk, or take your bike.

286

Taste something for the first time. Try a new veggie, fruit, or ethnic cuisine. Expand your food horizons instead of eating more and more of the same old thing, hoping it will taste like something else. Sometimes hunger can be confused with the desire for a new taste.

287

TIP OF THE WEEK	BUY NEW BRAS. LOTS OF THEM.

There are padded bras and minimizing bras; underwire and push-up bras; strapless, halter, and convertible bras; sport bras and side-supporting bras. Front-closure bras add convenience, cami-bras allow straps to peek out with style. There are smooth, seamless cups and exotic laces; sexy and sensible . . . The right bra, in the right size, can work wonders. Buy yours from a specialty store with professional fitters who know what does and doesn't work. Not only will the right bra eliminate bulges and strap lines, but it can distribute your "weight" in the most flattering way possible.

- To figure out your size, while wearing a bra measure around your body just below the bust and shoulder blades, and add five inches (if you get an odd number, round up by one). This is your *band size*. Next, measure around the fullest part of the bust, and subtract the band size from that. The number of inches difference between the two measures determines *cup size:* a one-inch difference is an A cup; a two-inch difference is a B cup; a three-inch difference is a C cup, and so on.

- Recognize the ill-fitting bra by bulges around it, puckers within it, slipping straps, shoulder furrows, a back band that rides up, or cups that runneth over.

- Recognize the inappropriate bra by whether you can detect the cup design under or see the bra itself through your blouse or sweater, or whether straps show.

- Call several better department stores in your area to schedule an appointment with a fitter. Ask about special "fit events," when manufacturers' representatives visit. Wacoal, for one, offers a computerized demonstration on its Silhouette Analyzer, which outlines your shape before and after you've been fit with a recommended bra style. See the difference the right style and fit can make.

288

Pass up patterned panty hose, and give dark-hued hose a good look. Patterns will stretch to emphasize your every curve, and even nonpatterned hose can distribute color unevenly (read: unflatteringly) on the leg if it's not a perfect fit. Opaque is more forgiving.

289

Match the color of your shoes to the color of your hose. Your legs will look longer and slimmer.

290

Expand your salad greens universe. The more interesting the flavor, the less boring the salad. Experiment with Bibb and Boston lettuces, romaine, radicchio, endive, frisée, watercress, arugula, even flat-leaf parsley. The more taste you put *in* your salad, the less you'll need to put *on* your salad in the form of fattening dressings and toppings.

291

Dip into chocolate instead of biting into chocolate. Cut your consumption by melting some down and dipping fresh, filling fruits like apricots into the sauce.

292

"Think Dumbo," and "fly" on your own. Remember Dumbo: Walt Disney's lovable cartoon elephant who could fly as long as he held a "magic" feather in his trunk, but later learned the ability was all within himself? The dieter's equivalent: "miracle" diet pills and herbal supplements that promise to have you losing megapounds. Look closely at the small print that accompanies them, and you'll find they all call for a sensible diet and exercise to work. Call it the Dumbo Feather Phenomenon: believing an item has magical powers that enable you to do something you can really do on your own. Save your money on the feather.

293

Have one now, have one later. Keep a sealable container on the table when you're eating, and for every forkful of food you eat, put another forkful into the container to be stored for another meal. If doing this would tempt you to have that other meal immediately, use a trash can as the "container," and write off the wasted food as a sacrifice for the cause.

The more time you spend on any one meal, the more filling the food will be. Plan at least twenty minutes for a leisurely breakfast, thirty minutes for lunch, and forty minutes for dinner, including between-courses breaks to breathe and digest. This doesn't mean you have to eat more; instead, chew slowly, chew thoroughly, put down your silverware between mouthfuls, sip a beverage between bites, and take the time to actually *taste* your food.

295

Dress in V's for victory. Clothing with down-pointing V-shape features—V necks, pointed collars and vests—guides the eye downward in a slimming vertical sweep. (All bets are off if any of those V's are bordered with ruffles.)

296

Lengthen round necklines. Round necklines make your face look rounder. If you do wear them, soften the look with a long necklace or a long, loosely tied, soft scarf to add a more flattering vertical effect.

297

Avoid turtleneck "spillage." Turtlenecks can be great for hiding double chins, but they can also create "spillage." Be sure the neck isn't too high or too tight to cause any part of your chin or neck to runneth over, and defeat the purpose.

298

Have a steaming bowl of low-calorie consommé, broth, vegetable soup, or a hot cup of decaffeinated tea before your meal. Not only will the soup or beverage itself be filling, but many people find hot foods quench hunger better than those that are lukewarm or chilled.

299

In the kitchen, before your meal, arrange one moderate-size meal's worth of food on your plate, and bring it to the table—to avoid repeated trips back and forth to the temptations of the stove, oven, and refrigerator, and keep from repeated dips into table-side serving dishes. When the food on your plate is gone, you'll know the meal is over. Period.

300

Tell it to a worry doll. Guatemalan legend holds that if you share a problem with a worry doll before going to bed and then place the doll beneath your pillow, by morning the doll will have taken your worry away. Tormented by chocolate? Having difficulty resisting dessert? Tell it to a doll and let *it* get fat. (Find the dolls at many museums, and on the Internet.)

301

Contrary to popular opinion, the most frightening Halloween sights are not the monsters, ghouls, or goblins that show up at the front door, but the inches that appear on your waistline and the numbers that appear on your bathroom scale afterward. Try these tricks:

- For trick-or-treaters, buy candy you don't like eating to reduce the temptation to eat it. Buy it *on* Halloween, buy it late in the day, and don't open the package until the first doorbell ring.

- Spend the evening at a good, scary double feature, and don't come home until all the tricking and treating is done. (Bring your own air-popped popcorn to the theater.)

- Instead of candy, give the inexpensive-yet-cool party favors or fun figurines available in the toy section of most discount and educational supply stores.

- Assign the trick-or-treat patrol to your husband or kids while you relax—far from the doorbell—with Stephen King.

- Buy a pair of fang false teeth and wear them all night. (No cheating!) You won't eat a thing.

- Assign another member of the household to disburse—and hide—any treats your own little tricksters bring home.

- The morning after, contribute every last bit of leftover candy to your office, your husband's office, or your kids' classrooms.

302

Perform an exorcism. Rid yourself of weight-loss demons.

Step 1. On individual sheets of paper, write out the things that bedevil your diet: leftovers, your mother's snide comments, chocolate. . . . (For that special "abracadabra" effect, we recommend silver ink on black paper.)

Step 2. Cast those nasty temptations out of your life. Shredding, burning, burying, and flushing all work heavenly well.

303

Try witchcraft. It's a law of nature that people who are struggling to lose an ounce tend to have partners and/or friends who can eat anything and gain nothing. Ask for a lock of their hair, wear it in a locket, and claim the power.

304

LEARN TO LIGHTEN YOUR POTATOES, AND YOU CAN LEARN TO LIGHTEN YOUR WORLD.

The average American eats 140 pounds of potatoes a year, according to the U.S. Department of Agriculture, making it the most popular vegetable in the country and, not coincidentally, a likely candidate for top culprit in our nation's obesity woes. The problem: Calling a potato a vegetable is akin to counting ketchup as one. The beloved spud contains enough starch to more than qualify it as a full-fledged carbohydrate.

Just as is true for most of our basic foodstuffs, however, most of the damage comes not from the food itself, but from the ways in which we prepare and dress it. Here are five yummy ways to cut back on the fat and calories so often associated with the spud. Use them whenever—and on whatever—you can.

Roast it: Replace fat-drenched french fries with lighter but no less tasty "french roasts." Slice potatoes into wedges, and either spray with fat-free cooking spray or, with a very few drops of oil on your hands, massage the wedges until lightly coated. Spray a baking sheet with fat-free cooking spray and arrange the wedges in a single layer. Season with salt and pepper, and roast at 450 degrees until brown (about twenty minutes on each side). Variations: Slice the potato into the fry shape of your choice; for "potato chips," slice the potato into thin disks and watch for burning. Worth trying with other veggies as well.

Nuke it: Puncture the potato, and microwave for ten to fifteen minutes (turning halfway through), then allow it to rest in aluminum foil wrap for a few minutes to cook through. Save hundreds of calories and fat grams by bypassing the butter and sour cream. Instead, top with chopped raw or steamed veggies that have been tossed with a low-calorie salad dressing, or some reduced-fat vegetarian chili and a sprinkling of low-fat shredded or grated cheese, or even some low-fat yogurt.

Steam it: New or red potatoes are great for steaming, and creamy enough to delight the taste buds with just a dash of pepper and salt.

Mash it: Cut baked or steamed potatoes into small pieces, and place in a large bowl. Toss in a cup of steamed cauliflower, turnips, or any other lower-calorie vegetable to bulk up the potato volume without bulking up the calories. Add just a dab of light butter or margarine; salt, pepper, and seasonings to taste; a splash of fat-free nondairy creamer; and mash until combined. Transfer into a casserole dish, cover, and reheat in a 350-degree oven, or for a few minutes in the microwave.

Mix it: For mayonnaise- (i.e., fat-) free potato salad, dice steamed potatoes and combine with just a teaspoon of good olive oil, chopped scallions, salt, pepper, and a splash of vinegar to taste.

305

Don't drive past the doughnut shop. That doesn't mean to stop at the doughnut shop, it means take a route that won't bring you within tempting range of it. Ditto: bakery and ice cream parlor.

306

While waiting in the supermarket checkout line, fend off the fattening impulse buys lurking near the cash register and calling your name. Keep busy by sorting through your coupons, rearranging your groceries, munching on some of the prewashed baby carrots in your cart, or gorging on those deliciously awful gossip magazines you'd never actually take home.

307

Hold in your stomach. Not only will it look flatter, but you'll be strengthening your abdominal muscles at the same time—a boon for your spine, which can suffer mightily from weight-related stress. Do it:

- When you climb stairs

- During television commercials

- While a companion is talking

- While you're watering your house plants

- Whenever your phone rings

- While you're waiting for someone you've phoned to answer

- While you're on hold on the phone

- While you're waiting in the supermarket checkout line

308

TIP OF THE WEEK	READY YOUR HOLIDAY DESSERT DEFENSIVE.

Let's not even pretend that skipping dessert at the big holiday meal is an option. But that doesn't mean you have to wave any white flags.

- Assign the dessert preparation to willing guests, and distance yourself from the whole process. Ask them to make something that presents you with the least temptation possible. Think fruit cake.

- Bake a lower-calorie, lower-fat version of a higher-calorie, higher-fat treat.

- Create a gorgeous fresh fruit salad to serve sundae-style over sugar-free, low-fat frozen yogurt. On a holiday platter, arrange orange slices that have been sprinkled with lemon zest or chopped ginger.

- Instead of a cake, bake apples.

309

Start a cooking-light library. Splurge on a basic set of really good low-calorie cookbooks with yummy pictures to remind you that nonfattening doesn't have to mean unappealing.

310

Do *not* tell your family you're feeding them from your low-calorie cookbooks, lest they not yet know that nonfattening doesn't have to mean unappealing, and try to convince you to cook fattening instead.

311

Don't spend more than five minutes reviewing a menu. The longer you look, the more likely you are to find a higher-calorie, higher-fat temptation. Scan the selections for what suits your diet best, make up your mind, and order before you can change it.

312

At a restaurant, have the waitperson package half your meal in a take-home bag *before* you start eating.

313

When resistance is futile, drop your dinner roll on the floor. Do it discreetly enough so it looks like an accident, but noticeable enough by fellow diners or dining companions to keep you from eating it after you've picked it up. Don't let the waiter or anyone else bring you a replacement.

314

Place your napkin over your food and press down on it to keep yourself from changing your mind after you've decided you've had enough of a meal. You won't win any table manners contests, but neither will you be likely to eat any more.

Having predetermined serving boundaries is worth the few extra cents you pay for the packaging, especially for those of us who are serving-size challenged, or who consider measuring cups and measuring spoons a personal affront. If you've ever jammed two cups of pasta into a one-cup measure, or skimmed the excess straight into your mouth, this means you. Premeasured portions will help keep you honest when you say, "I had only *one*."

316

Instead of a big holiday dinner, have a big holiday. Instead of centering the celebration around the table, cook up a menu of food-free activities. Look for a wide range of "recipes" in your newspaper's events calendar.

317

For elegant, leftover-free desserts, serve individual treats, like petit fours, fruit tarts, mini-cupcakes, individual custards, or single slices of something fabulous from the bakery. Buy one per guest.

318

Don't starve yourself on holiday mornings to "leave room" for the big meal. Instead, have a good, filling breakfast (a bowl of high-fiber cereal or a slice of toast, an egg or a scoop of low-fat cottage cheese, some fruit) to keep from becoming famished and out of control. If the dinner's later in the day, have a hearty bowl of soup or a healthy salad before you leave your house or guests arrive at yours.

319

Decide what to eat *before* you enter the kitchen. The less time you spend perusing your refrigerator and pantry, the less you'll be tempted by what's in them.

320

Do sushi. At least give it a try. It's fresh, it's lean, it doesn't come laden with sauces, and if you pile on enough spicy wasabi and ginger, you'll *have* to eat it slowly. Request reduced-sodium soy sauce, go easy on the rice, and ask to be seated in a private *tatami* room to protect you from the deep-fried tempura at the next table. For beginners, we recommend the (cooked!) shrimp, crabmeat, salmon, and tuna. Still scared? Have a vegetarian selection.

321

 Cut your sandwiches into quarters to fool your-self into thinking you're eating more of them.

322

 "Reduced fat," for instance, isn't the same as "low fat." The Food and Drug Administration and the U.S. Department of Agriculture say so. To be specific:

Reduced/fewer calories: 25 percent or less (calories or fat) than the traditional food

Light: One-third fewer calories and/or 50 percent less fat per serving than the traditional food

Fat free: Under 0.5 gram per serving

Low fat: 3 grams or less per serving

Low calorie: Under 40 calories per serving

Calorie-free: Under 5 calories per serving

Lean: Under 10 grams fat, 4.5 grams or less of saturated fat, and less than 95 milligrams cholesterol per 100 grams

Extra lean: Under 5 grams fat, fewer than 2 grams saturated fat, and fewer than 95 milligrams cholesterol per 100 grams

323

Close containers while they're on the table. Better yet, serve out your portion—of butter, dressing, ketchup, or whatever—and put them back in the fridge before you start to eat. You'll be less inclined to add more calories, and you *and* your table will both look better for it.

324

Eat just the black half of the black-and-white cookie. Have the white tomorrow.

325

Cut your salad dressing with a little extra vinegar and some water to cut fat and calories.

326

Allow yourself a splurge day once a month. Knowing a treat day is coming can help you resist temptations on all those other days. And if you skip the splurge, you get to feel that much more virtuous.

327

When you go to a restaurant, don't look at the menu. Keep tantalizing descriptions of meals out of your sight and they're more likely to stay out of your mouth. Think up a light and delicious selection before you arrive at the restaurant, and ask to have it prepared your (light) way. If your dining companion wants to hear the recitation of the evening's specials, excuse yourself. Out of earshot, out of mouth. And we won't even *talk* about the dessert tray.

328

Remember that there is no such thing as a free lunch. Attention, business lunchers: What you don't have to pay for out of your pocket, you will still have to pay for on the scale. Decide what it's worth to you.

329

TIP OF THE WEEK	USE CONDIMENTS, HERBS, AND SPICES TO ADD FLAVOR WITHOUT ADDING CALORIES OR FAT.

There *is* taste without heavy sauces. Try one new ingredient every week.

- *Pepper:* Black, white, it even comes in green. "Pink" peppercorns are a berry with a sweet peppery flavor. For heartier taste, buy whole peppercorns to grind fresh in a pepper mill.

- *Adobo:* An all-purpose seasoning popular in Latin cooking, it is often added to lemon juice or vinegar to make a marinade.

- *Mustards and horseradishes:* Smooth or coarse; hot or sweet; herb, wine, or garlic; mild Dijon to spicy Chinese. Use it on meats, in salad dressings, with cheeses, potatoes, or breads—wherever you want to add a little "oomph." Avoid the honey varieties, with heavier sugar content.

- *Salsa:* America's number one condiment has one-third as many calories as ketchup and three times the taste.

- *Old Bay Seasoning:* Shake the classic, superversatile Maryland spice onto steamed or broiled seafood, poultry, salads, meats, and vegetables.

- *Lemon juice:* Great on veggies, squeezed fresh from the fruit.

- *Blackened redfish seasoning or other blackening spices:* Heat a cast-iron skillet or the grill to red hot, rub the seasoning into your favorite seafood, and enjoy better-than-fried fish with an extra crispy, spicy crust, Cajun style. Caution: If you don't want your kitchen blackened, do your blackened cooking outdoors.

- *Ethnic flavorings:* From Jamaica's jerk spices to Japanese wasabi, there's a wide world of spices to explore. Check the ethnic foods section of your supermarket, or visit a specialty grocery store.

- *Hot sauces and Tabasco:* Give your taste buds a jolt.

- *Vinegars:* More than a great salad dressing, the variety of vinegars includes fruity apple cider vinegar, pungent red or white wine vinegars, mild malt vinegar, sweet balsamic vinegar, herb vinegars, fruit vinegars, rice vinegar . . . Use it in marinades, dressings, and sauces, or, with Old Bay Seasoning, on french fries. Avoid rich and sweet cane vinegar, made from sugarcane.

- *Soy sauce:* Not just for Chinese food, it makes a tasty addition to many vegetable dishes, sauces, and soups. Use reduced-sodium varieties.

330

Buy only one portion of a precooked meal at a time. That way you'll *eat* only one portion at a time.

331

Buy only one portion of dessert at a time. That way you'll *eat* only one portion of dessert at a time.

332

Buy one day's meals at a time. Not only will it cut down on overeating, but those additional trips to the market count as exercise.

333

Be buffet savvy. Being faced with table after table of unlimited food doesn't mean you have to *eat* table after table of unlimited food. But neither does it mean you can't have a delicious and filling meal. Start with a healthy serving of salad to take the edge off your hunger, then visually survey—without sampling—the entire spread to see what's being offered, and prevent a last-minute pile-up of the unanticipated yummies that always seem to hide at the far end. Add more greens to your plate before the next go-'round so there's less room available to fill with fattening foods. Choose three favorites, and enjoy a modest serving of each, before allowing yourself a sensible helping of dessert. Extra credit for jogging around the buffet table to work off what you eat.

KNOW HOW TO HANDLE A FOOD PUSHER.

They're everywhere. Well-intentioned (or not) family members, friends, and coworkers intent on getting you to "just have a bite." Face it: Not everybody wants you to look slim and svelte; you'll only make them look heavier. And even those who *do* have your best interests at heart have been brought up in the same "food means love" culture as you have. If they love you, they'll want to feed you.

Until such time as the food you eat "for" others ends up on *their* hips, arm yourself with a few sentences and strategies with which to respond without hurting their feelings, or causing you guilt. Anticipate challenges and role-play your responses with a *supportive* friend. (Don't tell your relatives we said so.)

- At family gatherings, do the words "Is there some-thing wrong with my cooking?" compel you to clean off your plate and ask for seconds? Try: "I'm so full I just can't eat another bite—but I'm not leaving without taking some home!" Have it tomorrow, or feed it to hubby.

- "Look at the cookies Jennifer brought to the office!" doesn't mean you have to *eat* the cookies Jennifer brought to the office. Say you'll take one for "later," and toss it into the circular file or, better, into the washroom drain while Jennifer and coworkers are otherwise occupied.

the little book of dirty diet tricks

- Is the passage of a serving dish down the table your family's "code" for "take a little more or there'll be trouble"? Pass it along, making "filled to the gills" moans, and sound enthusiastic as you ask for the recipe.

- Of course you want to support the neighborhood schoolchildren working so earnestly to raise money for a good cause. So when they come to your door selling their chocolate bars and cookies—or when their parents hawk them at your workplace—buy a package or two. And let them keep the sweets. Better for their cause *and* your cause.

335

Nonstick your kitchen. Equip your kitchen with a good set of nonstick pans and utensils that will more than pay for themselves with the money you'll save by not having to buy fattening butter and shortenings to grease them. Silpat, a reusable baking sheet liner from France, available at many specialty kitchen stores, even eliminates the need for flour. *Magnifique!*

| TIP OF THE WEEK | **KEEP A KITCHEN WISH LIST OF COOKBOOKS AND GADGETS THAT WILL HELP YOU COOK LIGHTER AND LEANER.** |

 When you're asked what you want for your birthday or a holiday, you'll be prepared. Like most gift requests: the more specific, the better—include brand names, colors, and sizes, when you can.

- Specialty cookbooks filled with light, ethnic, dessert, or vegetarian recipes

- A jazzy new food scale, and a set of measuring cups, to accurately weigh and measure portions

- A vacuum packer, to store and freeze individual portions of food

- A set of good knives, to slice the fat from meats

- Colorful disposable containers, for saving individual portions of leftovers, or sending them home with your guests

- A salad spinner, to make salads easier and faster

- A water filter—whether installed in your sink or on your refrigerator shelf—to clean out impurities and improve taste

- A fat-draining indoor griller

- A dehydrator, to transform fruits into healthy portable snacks that last longer than fresh

- Mini-muffin tins or loaf pans, to make portion sizes smaller

- A juicer, for fresh and healthy no-sugar-added refreshment

- Nonstick utensils, pots, and pans, to cut back on fattening oils and greases

337

Start an eating "advent" calendar. Children use advent calendars to count down the days to Christmas; you can use the same idea to count down the days to a reward of your own.

Step 1. Buy a calendar and a set of colorful stickers.

Step 2. Choose a treat—a movie, a new pair of earrings, a facial—as a reward for sticking to your diet. (Be specific about what "sticking to your diet" means—whether staying below a certain number of calories per day, or not eating between meals.)

Step 3. At the end of every day you're successful, place a sticker on the calendar. When you've placed stickers on seven consecutive days, reap your reward.

338

Start an exercise "advent" calendar. Choose a treat you'll give yourself for sticking to your exercise program—taking a twenty-minute walk, for instance, or riding your bike ten miles. On every day you work out, add a sticker to the calendar. When you've placed stickers on seven consecutive days, collect your reward.

339

Have a spritzer instead of a glass of wine. Have one part wine to three parts spritz, and think of the club soda or effervescent water as a drink-extender. A wine cooler—with about half the calories of its full-strength counterpart—is another option.

340

Ask the bartender to make it light. He or she will be more than happy to oblige. Watering down a drink out in the open is a lot easier than doing it behind the bar.

341

Pile on the rocks. Add as much ice to alcoholic drinks as can fit in the glass, and drink slowly enough for it all to melt before you finish.

342

Sip alcoholic beverages through a cocktail straw. The narrowness of the straw will slow you down. To slow down even more, bend the straw at a right angle.

343

TIP OF THE WEEK	USE DIET MIXERS.

Rum and Diet Coke. Gin and diet tonic. Alcoholic drinks contain a lot of empty calories. Conserve the calories you can.

MIXER	CALORIES PER OUNCE
Club soda, water	0
Diet sodas	0
Tomato juice	6
Ginger ale	9
Tonic	9
Cola	12
Orange juice	14

MIXER	CALORIES PER OUNCE
Pineapple juice	14
Cranberry juice	19
Cream	106

344

Don't even *think* about drinking so much that you'll be sick and expel all those calories. First: Bingeing and purging of any variety is extremely damaging to your health. Don't do it. Second: For all the wretchedness you'll be causing yourself, you probably won't expel all those calories anyway.

345

Keep a 911 treat box for munchy emergencies. In a securely closed container hidden in the back of an inconveniently high pantry shelf, keep an assortment of items that are all twenty-five calories or less, and reach for the box when the munchies strike. Remove up to five pieces (depending upon whether it's a five-treat emergency or a two-treater), put the box back, and very slowly enjoy one treat at a time until the emergency has passed.

346

Keep a 911 inventory for meal emergencies. Start a list of tried-and-true, fast-and-easy, hunger-stopping meals you know are satisfying, and keep the ingredients or products on hand for at least three of them: a serving of hearty bean soup (either from the can, or homemade and stowed in the freezer), a bag of prewashed-and-cut salad with light dressing, and a baking potato; a hamburger or veggie burger patty with a light, high-fiber bun, lettuce, tomato, onions, salsa, and pickles. And don't forget: Light, speedy frozen dinners are allowed!

347

Sit up straight. Grandma was right: Good posture is flattering and—if you hold in your stomach—flattening.

348

Buy a smaller size garment you're eager to wear, and "aim" for it.

349

Don't eat alone, especially when you feel susceptible to overdoing it. If you live alone, save the "irresistibles" you tend to overeat for meals you have with friends.

350

Shop until you drop those pounds. Yes, you've read it here. Shopping *can* be a legitimate weight-reducing technique. Need we bother to list the reasons?

- It keeps you away from the refrigerator. (But do bring along some healthy portable snacks to keep you away from the Great American Cookie concession in the mall's food court.)

- The money you spend is money you won't be spending on food. Extra credit for spending it on something that will help you with your diet.

- It's less costly than overeating. You'll save on the diet center fees, the gym fees, the bigger clothing costs, and the cost of the psychological counseling necessary to cope with Overeater's Guilt.

- Your household must need *something.*

- You must need *something.*

- It's physical activity. The steps you take getting around the store or circumnavigating the mall add up. If you take them energetically, they'll add up faster.

- If you buy smaller clothing, you can use it as motivation.

- The purchase of small gifts can reward your supportive friends and family members.

- The purchase of small gifts can reward—and motivate—you.

351

Relax with aqua therapy. The warm, relaxing water of the shower or bath—especially when scented with a calming aromatherapeutic fragrance—can quell even manic desires for forbidden foods. Plus, chances are your shower or bath is a safe distance from your kitchen.

352

Say grace before every meal and snack. Thank God or your favorite higher power for the food, and ask for help with your eating. Divine intervention *never* hurts.

353

Don't put out "fat food" for company. Every good hostess knows it's only right to put "something" in the snack bowls when company's coming, but you don't have to put out fattening foods that might lead you (or, for that matter, your guests) astray. Offer fat-free pretzels instead of greasy chips; a bowl of mixed nuts and a nutcracker instead of salted cocktail mix; fresh fruit and yogurt dip instead of candies. And when you're the guest, bring a lighter snack along as a hostess gift to keep yourself safe.

354

Hold the big holiday dinner at *your* house. You'll have control over what goes on the table—and what doesn't. Before the big day, prepare a menu of delicious, light holiday recipes, and stock up on a good assortment of food containers and a couple of pretty gift bows. As soon as dinner is over, fill those containers with leftovers, top each with a pretty bow, and send them home with your guests.

355

Be prepared for guests who ask what they can bring to the holiday dinner. Will you mind

having a high-fat spinach casserole on the table
right next to your low-fat version, or will you be
glad to provide an alternative for your guests?
Will certain dishes prove too great a temptation
for your comfort, or are you fine as long as you
took no part in its preparation? When in doubt:
Ask for flowers.

356

Do a "Kennedy." Instead of sitting around the
table after the holiday dinner, or collapsing in
the living room amongst bowls of nuts and
chips, gather up the guests for a game of touch
football, take a walk with a favorite cousin, have
a kite-flying contest, build a snowman, ride a
bike around the family compound.

357

TIP OF THE WEEK	MAKE IT A TEAM EFFORT.

Find a weight-loss partner. You'll get the combined benefits of a healthier, slimmer body, *and*
companionship along the way—something that
can make even the physical exertion of exercising more enjoyable. Other boons: Enlisting a
friend in your efforts gives you someone with
whom to celebrate your progress, and, by making a commitment to another person, you're less

likely to skip out on your commitment to the effort, and to yourself. Plus, you'll have someone with whom to share your orders at restaurants.

358

Use accessories to accent your best features and draw attention away from your weak points. The right earrings or hair ornaments, for example, attract the eye upward, and away from extra chins.

359

Wear the right hat for your head. Make sure your topper is in proportion to your body—neither mushroom nor pinhead is a flattering look. For a more slimming silhouette, let some neck show between the brim and your back.

360

Know how to handle a handbag. Big women shouldn't carry teensy handbags. And women with big hips shouldn't hang shoulder bags at hip level unless they want bigger hips.

361

Look at your eyeglasses. Like anything else you wear, they need to be the right size. Too small, and your face will loom large around them; too tight, and they'll cut into your skin. If you don't have contact lenses to wear while you're trying them on, bring along a sharp-eyed friend.

362

On thicker fingers and wrists, wear wider rings and bracelets. Or several narrow bands worn together. Delicate strands will only emphasize the heaviness of anything on which they're worn. And if they're tight enough to cause folds on your wrists, or make your fingers remind you of cocktail sausages, have the jewelry enlarged or replaced.

363

To thine own fashion style be true. Dress for yourself, not for this season's fashion runway. The toothpick-thin models who sport the latest designer whims might look good in trendy garb, but unless you, too, have been mistaken for a wire hanger, stick with classic looks that work. No matter how much hemlines rise or fall, or how broad shoulders and lapels become, the styles, cuts, and fabrics that flatter your figure won't change until your figure does. Another advantage: You'll be able to afford better-quality clothing if you don't have to replace your wardrobe every season.

364

TO THINE OWN SELF BE TRUE—AND DON'T LET SPOUSES OR SIGNIFICANT OTHERS HAVE YOU THINKING OTHERWISE.

At the risk of speaking marital heresy, we're here to tell you that there are some instances in which it really *is* okay to replace some of those "I do's" with "I won'ts." You do *not* have to eat like your spouse—especially if your spouse either (a) is headed down the very same overweight, unhealthy road off which you've decided to turn, or (b) is one of those annoying people who can eat whatever he wants without gaining an ounce.

Living with a person who requires gallons of chocolate-fudge-cookie-dough-ripple-chip ice cream in the freezer, a bevy of snacks and desserts in the pantry, and a kitchenful of other high-calorie repasts can present challenges on more than one level. If he is among those blessed with the eat-anything-gain-nothing gene, well, that's aggravating enough. But it gets worse. Not only do you end up facing temptation every time you enter the kitchen, but temptation can follow you to the after-dinner (read: front of the TV) locale, where your dearly beloved proffers "just a taste" in the name of connubial bliss.

"C'mon, have one little bite," he'll say, just like the snake said to Eve.

Take evasive action and arm yourself with your own low-calorie, low-fat alternatives, such as frozen yogurt or light desserts and treats, low-fat popcorn, shiny red apples . . .

365

CELEBRATE THE DISTANCE YOU'VE TRAVELED TO ENERGIZE YOURSELF FOR THE ROAD THAT LIES AHEAD.

Learning to drive, graduating from college, backpacking through Europe, planning a wedding, bearing a child, buying a house, landing The Job . . . Think of the many important and rewarding accomplishments of your life that you might not ever have dared to undertake if you'd agonized beforehand over the hard work and arduous details that were involved.

Losing weight is also hard work, and the journey can seem a long one. But this undeniable challenge can also be one of your greatest triumphs. Take credit for setting out on the journey, and celebrate every milestone along the way. Focus on the successful road you've already traveled, and you will find all the strength you need to keep moving ahead.

Take it one step, one pound, one inch, one belt notch at a time.

Index

About the Author

CAROLE BODGER has written for the *New York Times, McCall's, Glamour, Working Woman,* and *Longevity* and is the author of *Smart Guide® to Getting Strong and Fit, Smart Guide® to Relieving Stress,* and *Smart Guide® to Healing Back Pain.* A former New Yorker, she lives and stays slim with her husband and a small, but shapely, pack of Chihuahuas in Atlanta.